THE BALMIS EXPEDITION

THE BALMIS EXPEDITION

The Spanish Empire's War against Smallpox

DAVID R. PETRIELLO

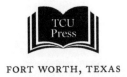

FORT WORTH, TEXAS

Library of Congress Cataloging-in-Publication Data

Names: Petriello, David, author.
Title: The Balmis Expedition : the Spanish Empire's war against smallpox /
    David R. Petriello.
Description: Fort Worth, Texas : TCU Press, [2023] | Includes bibliographical references
    and index. | Summary: "While the Spanish are often remembered for bringing
    smallpox and other diseases to the New World, little attention is paid to their efforts to
    eradicate one of the greatest killers in human history. In the middle of the Napoleonic
    Wars, King Charles IV funded and dispatched a humanitarian mission aimed at
    inoculating all of the imperial colonies in Latin America and Asia. Known as the
    Balmis Expedition, it was launched in 1803 and utilized Edward Jenner's new method
    to vaccinate people against smallpox. Using a human daisy chain of two dozen orphans,
    Dr. Francisco Balmis was able to bring the live virus across the Atlantic Ocean and
    later the Pacific. Yet, despite saving hundreds of thousands of lives, the history of the
    expedition was largely forgotten for the next 200 years. Many at the time resented the
    Scientific Absolutism that the mission represented, doing away with old methods and
    cures, as well as its economic implications. Finally, the onset of revolutions in the region
    only a few years later resulted in a rewriting of history which necessarily eliminated
    any positive accomplishments of the Bourbons. The Expedition became yet another
    victim of the Black Legend in Latin American historiography. A voyage which Jenner
    himself once called "an example of philanthropy so noble, so extensive," which served
    as the precursor for future world efforts at disease management, became forgotten. Yet
    despite this, its effects on the population and on public health efforts in the region were
    profound. The Balmis Expedition represented a perfect confluence of the tenets of the
    Scientific Revolution, the Enlightenment, and Absolutism, and bridged the divide
    between medieval and modern public health management"— Provided by publisher.
Identifiers: LCCN 2023036101 (print) | LCCN 2023036102 (ebook) |
    ISBN 9780875658575 (paperback) | ISBN 9780875658629 (ebook)
Subjects: LCSH: Balmis, Francisco Xavier de. | Jenner, Edward, 1749–1823. |
    Expedición Marítima de la Vacuna (1803–1810) | Medical expeditions—Spain—
    History. | Smallpox—Vaccination—Latin America—History—19th century. |
    Diseases and history—Spain.
Classification: LCC RA644.S6 P485 2023 (print) | LCC RA644.S6 (ebook) |
    DDC 614.5/210946—dc23/eng/20230907
LC record available at https://lccn.loc.gov/2023036101
LC ebook record available at https://lccn.loc.gov/2023036102

TCU Box 298300
Fort Worth, TX 76129

www.tcupress.com   *Design by Julie Rushing*

Dedicated to that iris that blooms and inspires . . .

In the Spring a livelier Iris changes on the burnish'd Dove;
In the Spring a young man's fancy lightly turns to thoughts of love.
—ALFRED, LORD TENNYSON

As well as to those brave historians who battle the Black Legend.

Contents

INTRODUCTION 1

CHAPTER 1 A HISTORY OF DISEASE IN SPAIN 7
Disease and Spanish History
The Health of the Habsburgs
Spain and Smallpox

CHAPTER 2 HEALTH IN NEW SPAIN 28
Disease and Exploration
Disease Treatment in Pre-Columbian America
Disease and Its Treatment in New Spain

CHAPTER 3 THE ENLIGHTENMENT AND DISEASE 43

CHAPTER 4 SPANISH EXPEDITIONS OF THE
EIGHTEENTH CENTURY 58

CHAPTER 5 JENNER AS JOHN THE BAPTIST 68

CHAPTER 6 SURGEONS, SMALLPOX, SOVEREIGNS,
AND ORGANIZING THE EXPEDITION 78
New Spain
Guatemala
New Granada
Bourbons and Smallpox
1802 Epidemic

CHAPTER 7   **BALMIS IN THE AMERICAS** 102
       Balmis Expedition

CHAPTER 8   **A RETURN TO CAJAMARCA** 128

CHAPTER 9   **BALMIS IN ASIA AND AFTER.** 143
       Aftermath of the Expedition
       The World's Response to Jenner and Balmis
       Scientific Absolutism and Latin American Revolutions

CHAPTER 10   **THE IMPACT OF THE EXPEDITION** 161
       Continuing Efforts in Latin America

CHAPTER 11   **DAMNATIO MEMORIAE** 181

       CONCLUSION 192

       NOTES 201

       INDEX 219

Introduction

ON SEPTEMBER 11, 1978, Janet Parker died at the Catherine-de-Barnes Isolation Hospital outside of Solihull, in England. Though she previously had been unknown beyond her local community, newspapers around the world carried the announcement in extended columns, often displacing other events on the front page. Parker's death was truly an extraordinary event, as she represented the last recorded fatality of smallpox on the planet. While working as a medical photographer for the University of Birmingham, Parker had contracted the illness through air ducts that connected her office to the lab of virologist Professor Henry Bedson. Bedson had been working with several virulent strains of the virus and had inadvertently allowed the illness to spread. Parker fell ill around the middle of August, though it would take over a week for her to be properly diagnosed and confined to an isolation hospital. Despite around-the-clock care, Parker succumbed to the illness three weeks later. Extreme measures were quickly taken to examine and isolate all who had come into contact with her. Both her parents were quarantined, with her father dying of an alleged heart attack and her mother successfully fighting off the illness, thanks to being treated quickly. Just as tragically, Professor Bedson subsequently cut his own throat, killing himself because of his involvement in the careless conditions that led to the misfortune.[1] Finally, the room in which Parker died was sealed off and left untouched for five years, serving as both a precaution against the spread of smallpox and a memorial to the last victim of this dreaded disease.[2]

Just under two years after Parker's death, the World Health Organization announced on May 8, 1980, that smallpox had finally been eradicated as a threat to humans. Centuries of efforts fighting against the disease, which culminated in an unprecedented twenty-year global campaign after WWII, finally had removed the scourge from the face of the planet. Janet Parker was the last victim of a disease that had claimed human lives for 3,100 years, a period of time that stretched back to Ramses V. With three hundred million dying of smallpox in the twentieth century alone, the destructive power of the disease dwarfed that of the two world wars and even the horrors of communism.[3] Donald R. Hopkins's sobriquet for smallpox, the Greatest Killer, was well earned.

Diseases have plagued mankind from the beginning, evolving alongside humans and expanding with them. As the Neolithic Revolution produced the growth of population centers, so too did it introduce endemic disease into this environment. Traditionally, early humans employed both religion and natural cures to prevent or drive off pestilence. Yet the continued presence and increasingly destructive impact of diseases over thousands of years shaped not only the history of humankind but also its institutions.

The presence of disease served as much as any other factor to drive the advent and expansion of civic government. Tribal rulers and, later, state leaders worked in conjunction with shamans and priests to appease nature and deities. Apart from an active concern for their subjects, these rulers sought to co-opt the influence of religious authorities in the management of disease to increase their own power and the power of their state. English and French medieval monarchs' claims to possess the inherent power to cure scrofula, Chinese emperors' ceremonies to prevent diseases, and even Henry Clay's call for a day of prayer and thanksgiving to avert the cholera pandemic striking America in 1832 are all examples of this process in action. The story of humanity's battle against disease is a tale that highlights the growth of science as well as the growth of government.

The decline in the power of the Roman Catholic Church and the rise in the power of the throne following the Protestant Reformation, the Enlightenment, and the Age of Absolutism saw similar growths in governmental interest in the prevention and treatment of disease. What was once viewed as falling within the bailiwick of God—through prayer or religious figures providing medical care—now became a field of activity for man and secular society. The contemporaneous onset of the Scientific Revolution also brought disease management into the realm of possibility. While Galen's millennium-old medical theories still held sway, new discoveries in the nature and treatment of disease were emerging.

This fits in well with Rudolf Kjellén's and Michel Foucault's ideas concerning the concepts of geopolitics and biopolitics. Both men pushed for the concept of a defined nation-state, with the health and well-being of its members being one of the primary concerns of the legitimate government. Attempts in the twentieth century by socialist and fascist states and Western democracies to perfect the health of their citizens through requirements and legislation are merely a continuation of this process. Apart from viewing their citizens' health as merely a paternalistic concern, leaders in the early modern period began to connect the health of their subjects to the economic prosperity and military strength of the nation. Frequent studies in the twenty-first century of the negative impact of smoking and childhood obesity are continuations of these trends.

Spain in the eighteenth century witnessed a sudden convergence of these factors that would lead to the Balmis Expedition, arguably the first attempt by a nation to confront the health of its citizens on a large scale. By the middle part of the century, the Scientific Revolution, the Enlightenment, and the notions of absolutism were all securely in place in Iberia. The combination of these three movements produced a notion of scientific absolutism: the idea of the state using science to enforce its goals. This new phenomenon could be driven by political, military, or strategic interests or, in keeping with notions of the Enlightenment and traditional Catholic mores, be motivated entirely by humanitarian concerns. Charles III of Spain, who reigned from 1759 to 1788, represented perhaps the epitome of this concentration of ideologies. Over the course of nearly three decades on the throne, he dispatched a number of botanical expeditions to various parts of the Spanish Empire. While ostensibly scientific in nature, these voyages also focused on issues of public health and on Madrid's political and economic interests in various parts of the planet. Scientific absolutism also sought to standardize the views of nature and the practice of science undertaken in the far corners of Spain's colonial holdings. Carolus Linnaeus's system of classification was often wielded as a blunt cudgel to unite the scientific thinking of the people as the Catholic Church united their spiritual thinking. Absolutism, be it scientific, political, or economic, bore mixed results for the Spanish Empire.

At the same time, individuals were making immense leaps in the field of medical science and public health. Edward Jenner, while not the first to discover the connection between cowpox and smallpox immunity, was able to spread knowledge of the practice of vaccination through his writing and persistence. Francisco Javier de Balmis, who had worked to treat outbreaks of the disease and other illnesses in both Spain and the New World, became interested in the topic in 1800, as soon as news of it reached the Continent. His translations of works by French authors discussing vaccination were some of the first to be published on the process in Spain. Yet it would take a perfect storm of occurrences for the Balmis Expedition to be launched, including a massive smallpox epidemic striking the Spanish colonies, the need for public and economic support during the Napoleonic invasions, the personal interests and pleas of Spanish viceroys, the Bourbon family's own heartbreaking experience with the disease, and the collision of the ideas of the Enlightenment and absolutism.

Despite its immense success, however, the expedition has been largely forgotten from the collective historical and cultural memory of much of the world. Balmis's triumph has been lost under the weight of the Black Legend and Latin American nationalism. Yet the expedition's preservation of millions of lives is worthy of record. Perhaps equally as important was its function as a perfect meeting point of so many philosophical, religious, and political movements. A king with the power of life and death, an attempt to challenge the inevitability of the grave, and a reliance on experimentation and reasoning, the ideas of absolutism, the

Enlightenment, and the Scientific Revolution were all brought together in the Balmis Expedition.

By the turn of the twentieth century, most developed nations were actively seeking to eradicate disease within their countries. Mass vaccination campaigns were launched as public health became not only a right but a responsibility. By the onset of the Cold War, the fight to eliminate pestilence had moved into Latin America, Africa, and parts of Asia. Under the auspices of the United Nations, global campaigns were developed to inoculate whole continents against some of the greatest killers of human history. Interwoven with notions of humanitarianism, economic concern, political necessity, and Cold War politics, these efforts closely paralleled those of Spain's King Charles IV. One of the greatest imitations involves the US President's Emergency Plan for AIDS Relief (PEPFAR). Launched under George W. Bush in 2003, PEPFAR used a variety of techniques and more than $80 billion to help save over a million lives in Africa.[4] Francisco Balmis and Charles IV began a two-century-long effort in the West aimed at eliminating world disease. In fact, the traditional narrative of public health efforts arising in England, or perhaps Germany, spreading to North America, and from there slowly infiltrating the underdeveloped parts of the planet is largely a myth in that it ignores these early Spanish efforts in Latin America that influenced opinions on the matter in the young United States and Europe.

This book will trace the role of disease in the development and history of Spain as well as of its colonies. A narrative will develop of a nation that was historically defined by illness. Likewise, the philosophical underpinnings of the expedition will be explored in an attempt to show that their roots were deeply imbedded in the history of both Spain and the Catholic Church. Finally, a thorough accounting of the aftermath of the voyage will seek to address the reasons the expedition's impact on subsequent public health campaigns has largely receded from the public memory. Balmis's philanthropic expedition was a product of many unique causes and represented a paradigm shift in scientific and civil practices.

CHAPTER 1

A History of Disease in Spain

I will punish that nation with the sword,
with famine, and with pestilence.

—JEREMIAH 27:8

CONTRARY TO THE PROPHET JEREMIAH'S preferred ordering of punishment, disease has killed far more humans throughout history than war or want has. In fact, disease was often a natural ally of war and want. Most major wars, up until the mid-twentieth century, saw more casualties from disease than from arrows, swords, or bullets. Disease decimated Germany during the Thirty Years' War, stopped Napoleon's invasion of Russia, and helped to drive General Cornwallis's British army from the southern American colonies. As late as World War I, more soldiers died from disease in the trenches than from the enemy's machine guns. Concurrently, three times as many humans perished on the planet from influenza than died in all the battles of the Great War. Likewise, famine bred sickness, which became the causative agent for most deaths during times of scarcity, such as Jamestown Colony's Starving Time and Ireland's Great Famine. Finally, even outside of war and famine, illness stood as the main cause of death throughout human history. Disease has always been the greatest scourge of humanity, and perhaps no pestilence was more feared or possessed a more storied history than smallpox. To understand and appreciate the launching of the Balmis Expedition, the role that disease, particularly smallpox, played throughout Spanish history must first be explored.

DISEASE AND SPANISH HISTORY

Spanish history, like every other nation's history, was intertwined with the presence of disease. Individual illnesses, local epidemics, and regional pandemics continuously directed the unfolding of events on the Iberian Peninsula since the Neolithic period. The pandemics that helped to bring down the Roman Empire, including the Antonine and Cyprian Plagues, almost certainly struck the Iberian Peninsula as harshly as they did the rest of the Mediterranean world. Their effects were one of the catalysts for the Germanic migrations that eventually overran the region, including the future lands of Spain. Likewise, the Justinianic Plague of the sixth century would have decimated the population of early medieval Hispania to the same extent it did other areas of Europe. Additionally, as nearly all warfare before the twentieth century was heavily affected by disease, the almost constant campaigns of the Reconquista saw many episodes of illness. Finally, the various monarchs and personalities that populate Spanish history saw their personal lives and political activities driven or limited by pestilence. Disease was a factor that shaped, drove, and delineated the history of the Iberian Peninsula.

The first major recorded epidemic to shape Spanish history was the Justinianic Plague in the sixth century. This early emergence of what is often presumed to be bubonic plague first appeared on the Iberian Peninsula in the year 541 and periodically returned to the region over the next century. An estimated 25 percent of the world's population succumbed to the illness over the course of a hundred years, perhaps fifty million people in total.[1] Historians have long surmised that the pandemic, in addition to causing massive loss of life, also helped to solidify the rise of Islam in the Near East and to facilitate its conquest of parts of the Byzantine Empire and North Africa.[2] This movement westward set the expanding Islamic Empire on a collision course with the Iberian Peninsula. As it is reasonable to assume that the Visigothic and Byzantine lands of Spain were equally devastated by the Justinianic Plague, the epidemic would have facilitated the Islamic invasion. This conquest defined the history of the peninsula for the next thousand years.

The next pandemic of importance occurred during the fourteenth century, at the height of the Middle Ages. The Black Plague arrived in Spain in 1348, most likely carried along the coastal trade routes from Genoa and Marseilles. The disease quickly overran Aragon. By 1349, the southern reaches of the peninsula, including Granada, had been breached as well. Despite the ongoing pandemic, King Alfonso XI of Castile launched a campaign in August of 1349 aimed at taking the fortress of Gibraltar. The importance of the promontory was demonstrated by the frequent sieges of it that took place between the various Christian and Islamic rulers of the peninsula during the fourteenth and fifteenth centuries. Alfonso's 1349 campaign to gain control of the fortress was the monarch's fifth such attempt to do so and seemed to promise the greatest chance for success. Coming on the heels of the Battle of the Río Salado, which had decimated the Islamic armies of Granada, the Castilian monarch felt confident in victory. However, despite his impressive host and determination, the Islamic garrison continued to hold out. Five months into the siege, the Black Plague struck the Spanish army, killing thousands, including Alfonso XI. As one chronicler recounted, "It was the will of God that the King fell ill and had the swellings, and he died on Good Friday, 27 March of the year of our Lord Jesus Christ 1350."[3] The Castilians were forced to abandon their siege and withdraw. Alfonso was the only monarch in Europe to succumb to the plague during its first great outbreak. Gibraltar itself would remain in Islamic hands for another century, before finally falling to the Spanish in 1436.

The loss of one Spanish monarch and the ending of a siege were not the greatest effects of the Black Plague. The disease caused an estimated 3.5 million deaths in the Iberian Peninsula and was particularly devastating in the urban centers and the island of Majorca, which lost 80 percent of its population.[4] Barcelona experienced a death rate of around 40 percent, and almost two-thirds of all clergy members there died. The high rate of death among the clergy was common throughout Western Europe.[5] Barcelona witnessed the typical chaos, breakdown of civic order, and rise of religious fanaticism that accompanied the pestilence in most European cities. Construction on most public buildings in Barcelona was halted, apart from churches, and Jewish residents of the city were frequently targeted. The El Call section of Barcelona was destroyed as residents feared that the Jews who inhabited the district had either physically caused the plague or else simply invited the wrath of God through their presence. Pedro IV attempted to keep order, but the almost total annihilation of the Council of One Hundred by the disease led to a breakdown in his ability to manage the population. In some areas of the region, serfs rose up and gained additional rights or economic opportunity, while in other areas, the landed aristocracy seized additional lands as peasant families perished.[6] The chaos and disorder that accompanied the pandemic would not be forgotten by political leaders in subsequent centuries.

Though the plague may have prevented Spanish power from expanding into Granada during this period, the epidemic aided in the preservation of Aragon. The Union of Valencia, an anti-royalist clique formed in the thirteenth century, had been battling to reduce Catalonia's power for several decades. By 1347, open conflict had erupted between the unionists and the royal court of King Peter IV. After several skirmishes and a failed attempt at a negotiated peace, Peter was captured and imprisoned. But the arrival of the Black Plague dramatically altered the situation in Valencia. Peter was freed from captivity amidst the unprecedented level of death and chaos caused by the disease. He quickly built an army and defeated the unionist forces at the Battle of Épila. The Black Death preserved royal power in Aragon, furthering the path toward Spanish unification a century and a half later.

The plague continued to ravage the Spanish peninsula periodically during the fifteenth century. Seville in particular suffered its effects in 1400 and again in 1410. The archbishop of the city, Gonzalo Mena Roelas, even fled from his seat in 1401 amidst the death and suffering, only to succumb to the illness a short time later. In Barcelona, the disease reappeared roughly every decade during the ensuing century, continuing to decimate the population. The outbreak of 1408–10 most likely led to the death of King Martin of Aragon. He had no surviving heir, and a short interregnum period ensued, ending with the ascension of King Ferdinand I in 1412 and the rise of the house of Trastámara, whose members would unite Spain at the end of the century. Outbreaks also occurred in Zaragoza in 1490 and 1495 and in Valencia in 1450 and 1465, and a rather large outbreak in 1485–87 struck Seville, Zaragoza, and Córdoba. The 1432 Lisbon plague was allegedly relieved through the work of the Dominican bishop André Dias. His success inspired the population and led to the adoption of the Holy Name Society in the city.[7] Overall, the various kingdoms of Spain saw little demographic growth during the fifteenth century because of the recurring ravages of bubonic plague, but the region did see certain political and social changes that eventually unified the region.

The Reconquista continued to be a prime catalyst for the spread of epidemic disease throughout the peninsula. For example, the siege and eventual conquest of Málaga in 1487 saw thousands of plague-infected prisoners of war brought into Córdoba. The outbreak that followed has been claimed to have killed up to two-thirds of the city's population, perhaps some fifteen thousand people.[8] Likewise, the other frequent sieges of major cities that dominated the centuries of war in Spain only rarely escaped eruptions of sickness, both among the soldiers within the walls of the cities and among those who surrounded the cities.

Attempts to prevent and combat illness tested the legitimacy of political and religious organizations for thousands of years. Historically, religious institutions had borne much of the responsibility for dealing with the outbreak of disease and had organized most of the responses to the Black Death in the fourteenth century. With the onset of the Renaissance and the slow-but-steady centralization of power in the hands of the monarchy, efforts by the state to both prevent and treat illness became more common. The 1408 outbreak of plague in Barcelona led to the establishment of a twelve-person plague board of health, one of the first to be established in Europe and a monumental step in the history of public health management.

Its responsibilities included effectively quarantining the infected and aliens, organizing charities, promoting medical services, and coordinating the removal of bodies.[9] Continuing this trend, Palma de Mallorca adopted the Ordinaciones del Morbo, which focused on quarantining ships arriving in the harbor from abroad.

Part of this trend in advanced public health management in later medieval Spain can perhaps be attributed to the higher level of medical knowledge inherent in the former Caliphate of Córdoba. In the fourteenth century, Ibn al-Khatīb famously speculated that the plague then striking Granada was transmitted from person to person, rather than caused by miasma or the will of Allah: "The individuals who have had contact with a plague victim will die, whereas the man who has had no exposure will remain healthy."[10] Though speculation exists that al-Khatīb was imprisoned and executed because of his unorthodox beliefs, as Islam officially viewed disease as a form of martyrdom, the Islamic world was certainly more advanced in public health management than the West was at the time.[11]

While Spain's geography allowed it greater access to the advancements of the Islamic world, it also served as the entry point of diseases into Europe. Typhus seems to have been one such illness that entered Europe through the Iberian Peninsula. Endemic to the Near East, the first definitive reference to the disease in Europe is usually attributed to the Spanish campaign to conquer the region of Granada in the 1480s. While besieging the Moorish capital, the Spanish army was stricken with lice-borne typhus. Over two-thirds of the army died of the disease, triple the number of deaths from combat. The bacterium was most likely brought to Spain by Spanish soldiers who previously had campaigned in Cyprus or the Near East. With the warfare, exploration, and trade that characterized the late fifteenth century, the disease soon spread across Europe, reaching England within twenty years. Typhus remained a constant on European battlefields for centuries, famously helping to destroy Napoleon's invasion of Russia in 1812. When Napoleon claimed that Spain was an "ulcer" in his empire, he may have in fact underestimated the region's biological role in his downfall.[12]

In 1505, the Black Plague once again descended on Iberia, ravaging the peninsula for over a year. This particular eruption of the disease became more notorious because of its aftermath than for its death toll. Outbreaks of disease and famine often led populations in Europe to seek scapegoats, with the Jews of the continent being the usual target of mob violence. In April of 1506, a Marrano, or converted Jew, was attacked and murdered after he publicly questioned a professed miracle at one of Lisbon's churches. A massacre ensued, and "in three days they slaughtered three thousand souls. They would drag and bring them to the street and burn them. They would throw pregnant women from windows and receive them on their spears, the foetus falling several feet away."[13] As King Manuel and most of the city's nobles had fled to avoid the pestilence, there was little that officials could do to calm the mob. Several thousand people lost their lives before order was finally restored. The government did its best to arrest and execute the leaders of the massacre, though this did little to prevent similar occurrences across the peninsula during future epidemics and undoubtedly fed into the politics of the Spanish Inquisition.

Shortly after the return of Columbus from the New World, a new and deadly epidemic emerged in Europe. Though the origins of syphilis remain a matter of debate among historians and epidemiologists, with some arguing for an American origin and others considering it a European illness, its impact has been well established. The disease appears to have first struck Barcelona in 1493, quickly spreading to other Spanish possessions.[14] The frequent movement of soldiers and sailors from Barcelona to Naples soon transferred the disease to that port as well. The contemporaneous French invasion of 1495, though accomplishing little in terms of political goals because of the outbreak of malaria in the region of Naples that decimated French troops, served to spread syphilis to the rest of Italy and France.[15] The disease's mode of transmission, its physical effects, and its ability to affect subsequent generations made it one of the most destructive and feared infections in Europe. Millions had already been infected by the disease when the writer Ruy Díaz de Isla opined,

> According to its loathsomeness I do not know anything to which I could more naturally compare it than to the serpent. For as the serpent is abominable, terrifying and horrible, so is this disease abominable, terrifying and horrible. It is a grave disease that separates and corrupts the flesh and breaks and rots the bones and disrupts and contracts the sinews.[16]

Syphilis not only devastated many individual Europeans but also helped catalyze more puritanical elements of the Protestant Reformation.[17]

Spanish soldiers seem to have likewise transported typhus to southern Italy, with the disease helping to prevent a French victory there in 1528. With the onset of the War of the League of Cognac, a French army under Odet de Foix descended on the Spanish-controlled city of Naples. After besieging the city, de Foix had the Bolla Aqueduct destroyed to worsen conditions for the defenders. But his actions proved to be his own undoing, as the ruptured pipes merely flooded the surrounding area where the French soldiers were encamped. Typhus soon broke out among the armies gathered there, killing thousands, including de Foix, and eventually forcing the French to withdraw. The failure of the papal-led league to oust the Spanish from the peninsula resulted in Habsburg domination of the region for two centuries. After the 1528 conflict, Pope Clement VII worked toward repairing relations with Charles V, a move that pushed the pope to deny Henry VIII's request for a divorce from Catherine of Aragon and began England's breakaway from the Church of Rome.

Disease was not always an ally to the Spanish during the sixteenth century, a truism demonstrated by the failure of the Spanish Armada. The sudden death of Álvaro de Bazán, the Marqués de Santa Cruz, in February of 1588 allowed King Philip II to appoint one of his court favorites, Alonso Pérez de Guzmán, the Duke de Medina-Sidonia, to command the fleet that the king was constructing to strike England. With little to no military experience, and purportedly habitually ill and suffering from sea sickness, Medina-Sidonia proved to be a very poor choice.[18] When the great fleet of over one hundred ships, eight thousand sailors, and eighteen thousand soldiers set sail in May of 1588, disease was already at work enervating its strength.

During the three-hundred-mile voyage from Lisbon to where the ships rounded Spain at Galicia, the condition of the crew was already rapidly declining. In June, Medina-Sidonia wrote to Philip II:

> Many of our largest ships are still missing . . . on the ships that are here there are many sick . . . these numbers will increase because of the bad provisions (food and drink). These are not only very bad, as I have constantly reported, but they are so scanty that they are unlikely to last two months . . . Your Majesty, believe me when I assure you that we are very weak . . . how do you think we can attack so great a country as England with such a force as ours is now?[19]

While Medina-Sidonia worked feverishly to upgrade and adequately supply the fleet's guns, the provisioning of food stores suffered greatly, especially with the rapidly expanding number of men tasked to the expedition, which grew from twelve thousand to nineteen thousand from February to June. Medina-Sidonia's subsequent decision to reduce rations during the voyage from Spain to the Netherlands would have only further promoted the outbreak of illness aboard the vessels by weakening his soldiers.

Though the weakened Armada certainly caused concern, disease at sea was not a new issue and certainly had been planned for by the Spanish. In fact, the increased number of troops aboard the vessels may have been added to anticipate this loss. Medina-Sidonia's operation bore another element. The Spanish fleet was set to dock in Calais and take on a battle-hardened army stationed in the Spanish Netherlands. Disease was also decimating the Catholic forces encamped there, with their overall strength falling from thirty thousand to around sixteen thousand. Even if the English had not ultimately driven off the Spanish Armada, it is doubtful whether this severely weakened invasion force could have accomplished its objectives.

The much-heralded English victory that followed in late July at Calais and Gravelines was not as absolute as remembered in popular histories. Sir Francis Drake's use of fire ships had not caused any significant damage to the Armada and had cost more English ships than Spanish ships. However, it had broken Medina-Sidonia's formation and led directly to the Battle of Gravelines. Though once again it was not an overwhelming tactical victory for England, Gravelines did produce certain instrumental strategic outcomes for England's Queen Elizabeth I. The anticipated linkup between the Spanish armies on the mainland and Medina-Sidonia's fleet did not take place. More importantly, it was now evident that the planned invasion would not occur and that the fleet was too weak from losses due to sickness and battle to risk a return voyage through the English Channel.

Medina-Sidonia decided to return to Spain to rebuild the expedition, but fear and necessity led him to choose a northerly route around the British Isles. Not only did he hope to avoid the English navy, but it was thought that the Catholic inhabitants of Ireland would readily supply food and supplies. The diseases that had plagued the vessels since departing from Lisbon had not abated, and they continued to devastate the crew. On August 11, the day after the Spanish began their long trek back home, Medina-Sidonia reported three thousand cases of typhus aboard his ships, which represented 15 percent of his total fighting force.[20] More men continued to succumb to fatigue and famine, and many of the fleet's horses had to be thrown overboard because of a lack of fresh water and food.[21]

Unbeknownst to the Spanish, a massive storm was heading toward the Irish coast, which ultimately destroyed the Armada. Not only did the wreckage of Spanish ships litter the beaches of the British Isles but so did the corpses of thousands of Spaniards. Many ships chose to land or ground themselves out of desperation for food and medicine. Because of their starving and disease-ridden condition, the crew of the La Trinidad

Valencera, which ran aground near Donegal, surrendered to the enemy rather than trying to fight or effect an escape. Unfortunately for them, the English chose to slaughter three hundred of the men. Another ship, the *Zuniga*, landed a force near Liscannor Bay to trade for supplies after eighty men aboard died of illness. Perhaps fearing English reprisal, the local Irish refused to trade with the Spanish, compelling the latter to resort to force of arms.[22] Finally, the ship *Nuestra Señora del Rosario* was captured shortly before reaching Calais, and its crew and passengers were confined at Torre Abbey in Torquay. In a building on the grounds known afterward as the Spanish Barn, the 396 men and allegedly a single woman were kept prisoner for weeks. The terrible conditions led to the outbreak of disease, and eventually many of the men and the young woman died.

In the end, two-thirds of Philip's great expedition died from disease and weather, rather than from English guns. Out of those several thousand men who did manage to make it back to the Iberian Peninsula, many succumbed to disease or the effects of malnutrition over the next several months and years, pushing the official death toll of the expedition even higher. The impact of illness was not lost on the Spanish commander, who placed much of the blame for the Armada's failure on disease. In the end, both weather and disease served to stop the Spanish invasion of England, saving not only Queen Elizabeth but also the Church of England. The much-repeated phrase about the Protestant Wind, "Flavit Deus et dissipati sunt," referred perhaps as much to the blowing wind as it did to the miasma of illness.

As can be expected, the English likewise were not able to escape from the diseases associated with the campaign. Typhus ran rampant on the returning English vessels and in the camps that dotted the coast. In July, a month before the Armada was driven back, Admiral Charles Howard, first Earl of Nottingham, reported sick lists for his ships that grew by the week. More English souls were swept away in the first weeks of the invasion by typhus, or gaol fever, than by Spanish gunnery. By the end of the year, over seven thousand Englishmen were in their graves as a result of the various pandemics that swept the British Isles. Howard memorialized the state of affairs in England in a letter to William Cecil in 1588.

> It is a most pitiful sight to see, here at Margate, how the men, having no place to receive them into here, die in the streets. I am driven myself, of force, to come a-land, to see them bestowed in some lodging; and the best I can get is barns and outhouses. It would grieve any man's heart to see them that have served so valiantly to die so miserably.[23]

The fleas and water of the English camps and vessels were far deadlier than combat.

In 1589, Drake was again tasked with leading an English fleet to Spain to destroy the remaining vessels of the Armada, provide aid to rebellious forces in Lisbon, and capture the Azores. With Raleigh's settlement of Roanoke only a few years before, clearing the seas and creating a line of communication with the Americas was vital to England's growth as a colonizing power. Launched in early 1589, the English Armada consisted of approximately 150 ships and 24,000 men. After successfully attacking La Coruña, Drake failed to take Lisbon and the Azores. Part of this failure arose from Drake's timidity during the campaign, which some historians attribute to his declining health. A few months previously, Drake had written, "Touched with some grief before my coming out of London . . . I have and do use all possible good means by physic following the advice of Doctor French; I do yet find little ease, for that my pain, not tarrying in one place, is fallen now into my legs and maketh me very unable to stand without much grief."[24] The English army was also crippled by disease both at sea and upon landing in Portugal.[25] By the time Drake decided to assault the Azores, there were very few men left healthy enough to man his ships. The expedition was ultimately a failure, with perhaps forty ships lost and close to 60 percent of the men dying, largely from disease.

Around the same time, diphtheria began to appear in periodic epidemics that swept across Europe. Spain alone saw six outbreaks of the disease between the years 1583 and 1638.[26] The eruption in 1613 was exceptionally deadly, with the entire year becoming known as *El Año de Los Garrotillos*, the Year of Strangulations. Reappearing periodically over the next two centuries, the disease proved particularly deadly to children. Deaths continued until the development of an antitoxin in the late nineteenth century, and included such notables as Princess Alice of the United Kingdom, US president Grover Cleveland's daughter Ruth, Prince Louis Charles of Prussia, and Princess Marie of Hesse.

THE HEALTH OF THE HABSBURGS

Individual bouts of physical and mental illness that struck members of the Spanish royal family also had profound impacts on the history of the nation. These illnesses not only directed the nation's course but also influenced the thinking of its various rulers, particularly those connected to the Balmis Expedition.

The unification of Spain, which is normally dated to the marriage and subsequent ascension of Isabella I of Castile and Ferdinand II of Aragon, occurred, in part, because of a series of personal illnesses. King John II, who ruled Navarre and Aragon from 1425 to 1479, frequently clashed with his eldest son, Charles of Viana. This opposition intensified to the point that war erupted between the two in 1451. At the same time, Charles's marriages promised little in terms of territorial gain for the kingdom. His sudden death from illness in 1461 brought his younger brother, Ferdinand, to power, allowing him to rise to the throne in 1479, following the death of King John.

A similar series of illnesses helped to place Ferdinand's future bride, Isabella, on the throne of Castile. John II of Castile was succeeded in 1454 by his third child, Henry. Two older children, Catherine and Eleanor, had died of illness just short of their second birthdays, making Henry IV the new ruler. The monarch proved unable to consummate his first marriage, to Blanche II of Navarre, while the paternity of the child from his second marriage was quickly called into question. More recent research has speculated that the king suffered from a pituitary tumor during his youth that, when combined with chronic kidney stones, would explain both his difficulty in producing an heir and his early death.[27]

Recognizing his imminent demise, Henry agreed to name his sister Isabella his successor and set about identifying potential suitors for her to marry. Despite Isabella's desire to wed Ferdinand of Aragon, Henry moved to force a marriage with Pedro Girón Acuña Pacheco, a master of the influential Order of Calatrava. Distraught, Isabella turned to prayer, only to have Pedro suddenly fall ill and die on his way to the capital. Though the marriage had been prevented, it created a rupture between the siblings. Two years later, John of Castile's only other surviving son, Alfonso, succumbed to the plague at the age of fourteen. Henry had little choice but to name Isabella as his heir. She was now free to marry Ferdinand in 1469. Because of their consanguinity, Cardinal Rodrigo Borgia produced a forged papal bull from Pope Pius II to allow the union. Interestingly, the pope had actually died five years previously of an acute fever, but the ruse went unnoticed.[28] With the subsequent death of King Henry IV in 1474, the throne of Castile passed to his sister, allowing for the unification of Spain under Ferdinand and Isabella.

Five surviving children were born to the first monarchs of a united Spain, though illness once again drastically affected their future. Their eldest child, Isabella, Princess of Asturias, was born in October of 1470. Following an initial marriage in 1490, which soon ended in the death of her husband, Isabella was wed in 1497 to Manuel of Portugal. Marriage to the crown prince of the nation seemed to promise the final unification of the entire Iberian Peninsula, a goal for many of its rulers since the fall of the Visigothic kingdom. A year later, Isabella gave birth to a son, Miguel da Paz, seemingly further cementing the nations together. But disaster soon struck the royal family. Isabella died shortly after giving birth, and her son succumbed to illness before his second birthday. Spain and Portugal would remain two distinct nations.

Isabella of Castile gave birth to her only surviving son, John, in June of 1478. Despite a promising marriage to Margaret of Austria, the eldest daughter of Emperor Maximilian I, John would never see the throne of Spain. Frail throughout much of his later life, John succumbed to tuberculosis in 1497. Margaret delivered a stillborn girl two months later and subsequently returned to Austria.

The deaths of Isabella and Ferdinand's other children left Joanna as the heir to the throne of a united Spain. She had been married at the same time as her brother in an attempt to solidify the nation's alliance with the Habsburgs. Joanna's husband, Philip I, would eventually bring the Netherlands, Burgundy, and the Habsburg possessions in Germany to the Spanish crown, bringing Spain into the politics of Central Europe in the sixteenth and seventeenth centuries. Following the death of her mother in 1504, Joanna became the titular ruler of Castile. Ferdinand refused to accept the new arrangement and capitalized on Joanna's absence and lack of interest to secure his own rule over both kingdoms. To legitimize his rule, Ferdinand claimed that Joanna was suffering from a mental illness. Joanna and her husband, Philip, returned to Spain in 1506, and civil war soon threatened to erupt between father and daughter. Interestingly, while Ferdinand quickly agreed to restore Joanna to power, Philip suddenly seized on her purported illness to make himself the ruler of Castile.[29] War between the two monarchs was averted in September of 1506 when Philip I died suddenly of typhoid.

Joanna's alleged madness was employed once more by Ferdinand to again deprive her of her power from 1506 to 1516. Only a year after the death of the king of Aragon, Joanna's son Charles arrived in Spain and likewise employed his mother's illness to make himself the sole authority in Castile. The rest of Joanna's life was spent largely in exile and isolation, with her condition slowly deteriorating until her death in 1555. Debate has existed since the sixteenth century as to the existence, nature, and extent of Joanna's mental illness.[30] Theories about her illness ranged from the idea that it was only a ploy by Ferdinand and Philip to wrest control of Castile from her to it being some form of inherited schizophrenia or the result of her ill treatment and isolation. The exact nature of her illness matters less to history than does the impact it had on the direction of Spanish politics.

Consanguineal marriages and inherited illnesses plagued the Habsburg dynasty for the next two centuries. Signs of these issues emerged almost immediately, with Charles I, who ruled over a vast global empire that included Spain, the Holy Roman Empire, the Spanish Netherlands, much of Italy, and the New World and who suffered from an enlarged jaw, gout, and epilepsy. The emperor's gout, combined with an outbreak of illness among his soldiers, even served to deliver him a crushing defeat at the siege of Metz in 1552.[31] In 1558, at the age of fifty-eight and stricken with such severe gout that he had to be carried around in a chair, Charles contracted malaria and died shortly afterward.[32]

His son, Philip II, was generally healthy, living to the age of seventy-one, at which point he died of cancer. Though he escaped the ravages of disease himself, Philip II's various wives and children were not so lucky. Philip was married four times and produced at least eight children who survived birth. His first wife, Maria Manuela of Portugal, gave birth to a son, but she died a few days later from complications. The boy, Carlos, would live to only twenty-three and died in 1568. Carlos seems to have suffered from a mental illness similar to Joanna's and was eventually imprisoned by his father.

Philip's second marriage, to Queen Mary of England, resulted in a successful pregnancy shortly afterward. Throughout much of 1554 and early 1555, both the English and Spanish realms anxiously awaited the birth of an heir. As the anticipated date for the delivery approached, Mary withdrew into her chambers and celebrations began in the streets of London, as rumors of a birth quickly spread. As the weeks went by it became increasingly apparent that Mary not only was not going to give birth but probably had never been pregnant. She seems to have suffered an episode of pseudocyesis, better known as phantom pregnancy. A few weeks later, as the size of Mary's stomach began to subside, her depression and melancholy increased. Mary almost certainly blamed the continued existence of Protestantism within the nation for her inability to become pregnant—God's divine punishment for the toleration of heresy. Over the next two years, her condition only worsened. Periods of depression alternated with headaches, fever, pain, and dropsy. By late 1558 she was largely blind, had lost her eyebrows, and was confined to bed, finally passing away on November 17.

Several possible causes have been suggested for the health problems, false pregnancy, and early death of Queen Mary. Ovarian cysts, fibroid tumors, uterine cancer, or a prolactinoma pituitary tumor seem to be the likely candidates. The last is a condition that produces false pregnancies, hypothyroidism, and the numerous other symptoms experienced by Mary during her lifetime. At the same time, Mary's inability to conceive may have been connected to her acquisition of Kell-positive genes from her father, Henry VIII, who suffered from similar reproductive issues.[33]

Philip's third marriage was to his cousin, Elisabeth of Valois, and it produced five children, of whom two daughters survived. Elisabeth herself died shortly after delivering the last child in 1568. Philip's final marriage, to Anna of Austria, also resulted in five children, of whom only one survived. The rest of their children died before the age of eight, including Charles, who succumbed to dysentery at the age of two, and Diego, who fell victim to smallpox at the age of seven.

Perhaps because of generations of consanguine marriages combined with poor medical practices, the Habsburg family continued to experience high infant mortality rates at the turn of the seventeenth century. Philip III and Margaret of Austria gave birth to eight children, three of whom died young. Philip's son Philip IV produced nine children with Elisabeth of France, only two of whom, Balthasar and María Teresa, survived into adolescence. The former was duly crowned Prince of Asturias, only to die of smallpox at the age of sixteen. Philip IV's subsequent marriage to his niece, Maria Anna of Austria, witnessed the birth of five children, two of whom died within a year of being born. His daughter, Margaret Theresa, married Leopold I of the Holy Roman Empire and produced six children, only one of whom lived. She died at the age of twenty-one. Philip IV was thus left with only two male heirs, Philip Prospero, who died at the age of four from epileptic shock, and Charles.

Charles would go on to define the illnesses related to close marriages that plagued the Habsburg court. Charles II grew up with severe developmental problems, delayed in both speaking and walking. Among his many health problems, it has been suggested that he suffered from pituitary hormone deficiency and distal renal tubular acidosis.[34] The former condition would help to explain the infertility that plagued him over the course of two marriages. Despite his severe mental and physical ailments, Charles survived until the age of thirty-eight, dying in November of 1700. His autopsy recorded that his body "did not contain a single drop of blood; his heart was the size of a peppercorn; his lungs corroded; his intestines rotten and gangrenous; he had a single testicle, black as coal, and his head was full of water." More recent speculation has arisen that he also suffered from either Klinefelter or Fragile X syndrome.[35] Regardless of the cause of his illnesses and death, Charles II's demise led to a succession dispute that plunged Spain and most of Europe into war that lasted until 1714.

Disease drove and limited Spain's accomplishments for centuries. Nowhere was this more evident than within the royal family itself. Illnesses, both genetic and acquired, ensured the union of Spain, prevented a permanent union with Portugal, ended the reigns of monarchs, caused succession crises, and ultimately led to the fall of the Habsburgs. Yet, of all the plagues that affected Spain and its history, none was more deadly or feared than smallpox.

SPAIN AND SMALLPOX

Smallpox has a long history, closely intertwined with the rise of civilization. Various theories exist as to the exact origin of the disease, with more recent genetic research placing it in East Africa around four thousand years ago.[36] As a member of the *Orthopoxvirus* genus, smallpox evolved along with a series of other viruses that included camelpox, cowpox, horsepox, and monkeypox. From there, it slowly spread out, crossing into the

Middle East and India before reaching East Asia. The illness seems to have spread in epidemic waves, often carried by invaders into eastern and western empires. China appears to have first encountered the illness during its dealings with the Xiongnu people of modern-day Mongolia, while the disastrous Antonine Plague that beset the Roman Empire in the second century most likely moved west with soldiers returning from a campaign against Parthia. War and the movement of soldiers appears to have spread the disease to Europe in 580. A possible outbreak among Ethiopian soldiers besieging Mecca in 569 seems to have been passed on to Byzantine troops, who then carried it to Italy a few years later. The Arab conquest of Spain most likely permanently introduced the illness into the region, and Crusaders from central and northern Europe took the disease home with them in the eleventh and twelfth centuries. All of these were most likely outbreaks of variola minor, with the deadlier strain only evolving sometime between AD 400 and 1600 in Asia.[37]

The "speckled" disease is spread by a brick-shaped virus called *variola*. Two forms of the infection exist: variola major and variola minor. Once either enters the body, humans experience a 50 percent chance of infection and remain most contagious during the first few days of contact. Usually, nine days will pass with few signs or symptoms of the disease, allowing the victim to unknowingly spread the virus to others. A fever, headache, and chills then follow as a rash slowly begins to develop on the body. Over the course of the next several days, pustules start to erupt on the skin and sores develop in the mouth and throat. It is from these symptoms that the disease acquired its various regional names. The internal effects of the virus produce the most harm, and in rare cases of black smallpox, hemorrhaging occurs, which almost certainly kills the victim. The disease normally runs its course in about three weeks, producing a mortality rate of around 25 percent. Variola minor was a much-reduced version of the disease that led to a less severe outbreak and fewer casualties.

Spain's experience with smallpox began earlier than it did for most other European countries. Even if the various episodes of the disease in the ancient world described earlier were actually outbreaks of smallpox, they were most certainly isolated epidemics. The Arab conquest of the Iberian Peninsula most likely would have introduced endemic variola minor to the region, well before it reached the rest of Europe. Tradition held that in 710, Roderick, the last Visigothic king of Spain, raped the daughter of a local lord, Count Julian. In revenge, the count supported the subsequent Arab invasion of the peninsula, which brought not only Islam but also smallpox to Western Europe.[38] As with typhus and, much later, syphilis, the Iberian Peninsula served as a gateway for disease into the rest of the Continent.

The fractured nature of the peninsula and the warfare associated with the Reconquista made disease a frequent occurrence in Spanish history. Repeated waves of bubonic plague and endemic smallpox affected the Iberian Peninsula and its history from the fourteenth to the sixteenth centuries. Yet the variola minor strain that inhabited Spain was often considered by medical experts at the time to be less of a cause of concern than bubonic plague. Against the latter, Alonso de Chirino recommended only prayer and flight, while for smallpox he laid out practical methods of avoidance and treatment.[39] Ruy Diaz de Isla, who famously lamented the arrival of syphilis, confirmed the common occurrence of smallpox during the fifteenth century by recounting in amazement that an acquaintance of his had never had the illness.[40]

The arrival of variola major sometime in the sixteenth century drastically increased the deadliness of outbreaks. The disease is estimated to have killed around four hundred thousand a year in eighteenth-century Europe alone. Because of smallpox's deadly nature, it is not surprising to see the rise of a saintly cult around the illness. Saint Nicasius, who was martyred by the Huns around 407, is said to have survived the illness and much later became the patron saint of those suffering from it. Though the addition of smallpox to his personal story is most likely a later component, he became a popular figure during the time the disease ravaged Europe. A devotional prayer to the saint ran so:

In the name of our Lord Jesus Christ, may the Lord protect these persons and may the work of these virgins ward off the smallpox. St. Nicaise had the smallpox and he asked the Lord [to preserve] whoever carried his name inscribed. O St. Nicaise! Thou illustrious bishop and martyr, pray for me, a sinner, and defend me by thy intercession from this disease. Amen.[41]

As the seventeenth and eighteenth centuries progressed, the bubonic plague gradually reduced its physical and psychological hold on Spain. In its place, this newer and deadlier form of smallpox began to decimate the population. It was to be this version of the illness that laid low the Spanish court, killed hundreds of thousands over several centuries, and inspired the launching of the Balmis Expedition.

Overall, genetics and geography were the directing factors of the path of disease through Spanish history. The marriage habits of the Trastámara and Habsburg dynasties led to the proliferation and worsening of certain genetic disorders. At the same time, Spain's unique geographic location led to both the influx of disease and medical science from the Maghreb region and the Near East and the export of illness to the rest of Europe and the Americas.

CHAPTER 2

Health in New Spain

A pestilence seized them, characterized by great pustules,
which rotted their bodies with a great stench, so that
their limbs fell to pieces in four or five days.

—DIEGO DE LANDA,
SIXTEENTH CENTURY

THE NEW WORLD, before the arrival of Columbus, was hardly a disease-free paradise. While Europeans and Africans certainly introduced diseases that decimated the Indigenous populations, bacteria and viruses predated their arrival. Likewise, many of the atrocities attributed to the Spanish by the Black Legend have now been thoroughly debunked. The vast loss of life that occurred after 1492 in the Americas can now be rightfully attributed to a microbial invasion rather than solely to the guns or swords of the conquistadors. It is a historical truism that disease existed in the New World before the arrival of the Spanish, serving to drive events and devastate populations. The introduction of new contagions in the sixteenth century merely increased this process exponentially.

DISEASE AND EXPLORATION

Biological evidence points to the existence of numerous diseases in the New World prior to the arrival of the Spanish. As well, the presence of deities among the Maya, Aztec, Inca, and other peoples whose bailiwick was the realm of illness certainly hints at disease as an object of concern for the Amerindians. Apart from such common illnesses as colds and degenerative conditions such as anemia and osteoarthritis, it's believed that tuberculosis, herpes, bartonellosis, typhus, and several other contagions existed in parts of the Americas.[1] But the low level of development among the Indigenous population, the north-south axis of the continent, and more localized trade meant that far-reaching epidemics were probably rare. Despite this, it is safe to argue that Indigenous peoples were not living in the germ-free paradise often associated with them. The Aztec *Annals of Cuauhtitlan*, in fact, recorded two major epidemics in the century preceding the arrival of Cortés.[2]

The entrance of Hernán Cortés into Tenochtitlán in 1519 and the sojourn of the Spanish there for a year undoubtedly introduced contagions into the capital. Following their expulsion in La Noche Triste (the Sad Night), the Europeans retreated to the coast, convinced that their chance to seize the capital had failed. Reports soon reached Cortés that a virulent outbreak of smallpox was ravaging Tenochtitlán. Well over 25 percent of the city's population succumbed, including the new emperor, overwhelming the civic authorities and resources of the city. Houses were simply demolished with the dead inside, and unclaimed corpses floated among the chinampas. The subsequent assault by the Spanish and their Indigenous allies in the spring of 1521 magnified the horrors within the town. "The ground and lake and fighting platforms were all full of dead bodies; they smelled so bad that there was no man who could bear it . . . and even Cortés was sick from the stench that penetrated into his nostrils."[3] By August of 1521, the city had fallen, and Cortés's allies rampaged through the deserted and devastated streets, enslaving or evicting those who remained. The great city of Tenochtitlán had fallen as much through pestilence as through force of arms.

Despite the fall of the Aztec capital, millions of Nahua peoples in various tribes and kingdoms still inhabited Mesoamerica. Disease once again aided the Spanish conquest, this time in the guise of the mysterious *huey cocoliztli*.[4] Striking between 1545 and 1576, the illness was recorded by several Spanish eyewitnesses. Fray Juan de Torquemada, the famed Jesuit scholar who was active in New Spain from the 1560s to 1624, recorded the following regarding the outbreak of 1576:

In the year 1576 a great mortality and pestilence that lasted for more than a year overcame the Indians. It was so big that it ruined and destroyed almost the entire land. The place we know as New Spain was left almost empty. It was a thing of great bewilderment to see the people die. Many were dead and others almost dead, and nobody had the health or strength to help the diseases or bury the dead. In the cities and large towns, big ditches were dug, and from morning to sunset the priests did nothing else but carry the dead bodies and throw them into the ditches without any of the solemnity usually reserved for the dead, because the time did not allow otherwise. At night they covered the ditches with dirt. . . . It lasted for one and a half years, and with great excess in the number of deaths. After the murderous epidemic, the viceroy Martin Enriquez wanted to know the number of missing people in New Spain. After searching in towns and neighborhoods it was found that the number of deaths was more than two million.[5]

The outbreak resulted in an estimated six to twelve million deaths in 1545, with perhaps an additional four million in 1576. Taken together, these numbers dwarf the estimated eight million inhabitants of Mexico who died from the smallpox outbreak spread by Cortés's men in 1520. The Spanish pacification and settlement of Mesoamerica was aided by this precipitous loss of life.

The exact nature of huey cocoliztli has been the subject of historical and scientific debate. For centuries it was assumed to have been smallpox, but contemporaneous accounts of the pestilence do not conform to the typical clinical picture of that disease. Francisco Hernández, the court-appointed physician-in-chief for New Spain in the sixteenth century, recorded his views on the outbreak.

The fevers were contagious, burning, and continuous, all of them pestilential, in most part lethal. The tongue was dry and black. Enormous thirst. Urine of the colors sea-green, vegetal-green, and black, sometimes passing from the greenish color to the pale. Pulse was frequent, fast, small, and weak—sometimes even null. The eyes and the whole body were yellow. This stage was followed by delirium and seizures. Then, hard and painful nodules appeared behind one or both ears along with heartache, chest pain, abdominal pain, tremor, great anxiety, and dysentery. The blood that flowed when cutting a vein had a green color or was very pale [and] dry. . . . In some cases gangrene . . . invaded their lips, pudendal [genital] regions, and other regions of the body with putrefact members. Blood flowed from the ears and in many cases blood truly gushed from the nose. Of those with recurring disease, almost none was saved. Many were saved if the flux of blood through the nose was stopped in time; the rest died. Those attacked by dysentery were usually saved if they complied with the medication. The abscesses behind the ears were not lethal. If somehow their size was reduced either by spontaneous maturation or given exit by perforation with cauteries, the liquid part of the blood flowed or the pus was eliminated; and with it the cause of the disease was also eliminated, as was the case of those with abundant and pale urine. At autopsy, the liver was greatly enlarged. The heart was black, first draining a yellowish liquid and then black blood. The spleen and lungs were black and semi-putrefacted . . . the abdomen dry. The rest of the body, anywhere it was cut, was extremely pale. This epidemic attacked mainly young people and seldom the elder ones. Even if old people were affected they were able to overcome the disease and save their lives.[6]

Dr. Hernández's description of the disease hints at a tropical hemorrhagic fever more than it does a traditional European illness. Many arenaviruses do exist in the New World, including Bolivian, Argentinian, Brazilian, and Venezuelan hemorrhagic fevers. Their lethality is demonstrated by the fact that several were chosen by the US government for use in its biological weapons program during the Cold War. With mice serving as their vectoring agents, the pestilence could have easily found its way into large urban population centers, especially as civic order and public sanitation broke down during the Spanish conquest.

A more recent genetic study, relying on the analysis of DNA from the teeth of victims buried in mass graves, has pointed toward a different type of illness. The vast majority of the remains tested positive for *Salmonella enterica*. The bacterium produces an enteric fever in its victims, similar in effects to typhoid. High fevers, vomiting, and rashes would have been hallmarks of the epidemic, all of which were reported by Hernández and Torquemada. Though the same bacteria have been found in the remains of a medieval body in Europe, it's still unknown if it was a European illness or if it was present in the New World before the arrival of the Spanish.[7]

Historical studies have revealed that the population of Mexico and Central America fell from a peak of around twenty million in 1520 to around only one million a hundred years later, in 1619. While the initial smallpox epidemic begun by the followers of Cortés in Tenochtitlán has been argued to have claimed eight million lives, the additional eleven million-plus deaths over the course of the following century were largely assumed to have been the result of other diseases, usually unidentified or simply blamed on the brutality of the Spanish. Yet, once the outbreaks of 1545 and 1576 are examined, a much deadlier epidemic than the smallpox wave of 1520 emerges. Further showing that the two later occurrences of illness were actually a new strain, the mysterious outbreak recorded by the Spanish in 1545 bore an estimated 80 percent mortality rate, while that of 1576 produced a 45 percent death toll.[8] This pattern would be typical of a first-time encounter with a new pestilence rather than of a re-eruption of smallpox.

The presence of preexisting large-scale epidemics is further evidenced by the Inca conquest of Chile, which was attributed by ancient sources to an outbreak of typhus. According to Felipe Guáman Poma, in his seventeenth-century *Chronicle*, the Inca were able to conquer the region of Chile during the reign of Pachacuti Inca Yupanqui "by the ravages of plague . . . disease and famine, even more than force of arms brought about the downfall of the Chileans."⁹ This strikingly foreshadows the fate of the Inca themselves almost a century later.

The Spanish encounter with the Inca in South America followed a similar path of confrontation and disease. In 1527, the grandson of the Inca empire's founder sat securely on his throne. Huayna Capac had done his own part to further expand the empire, stretching it as far south as Chile and Argentina. When news arrived that a foreign group had landed in modern-day Colombia, the emperor quickly proceeded north with a sizeable force. Though Huayna Capac never encountered the Spanish directly, he did fight several local tribes before returning home with much plunder. It appears that the Inca army also brought back an illness in their baggage train: possibly smallpox or bartonellosis.¹⁰ Regardless of the precise pathogen, by the end of 1527, the emperor, his heir, Ninan Cuyochi, and over a hundred thousand others had died. The disaster of this episode was that without a clear line of succession to the throne, civil war soon erupted between the remaining sons of Huayna Capac. A vicious internecine war raged from 1529 to 1532 between Huáscar and Atahuallpa. By the end of the struggle, a sizeable percentage of the empire's population had been killed. Fields were ruined, villages depopulated, loyalties questioned, and an empire built on conquest and enslavement was beginning to show cracks. It was at this precise waning of power that the Inca engaged Francisco Pizarro's army in 1532 at the famed field of Cajamarca. The more traditional history, which blames either the Spanish or smallpox for the destruction of the Inca, should be rewritten to account for "the demographic disaster [of] three decades of near total war, excessive labor demands, wholesale environmental destruction, widespread famine, and sheer cruelty. Alien diseases [were] secondary factors, dating from 1558 with the first smallpox epidemic, once the population has already been halved."¹¹

Similar incidents occurred throughout the Americas as Europeans first came into contact with Indigenous peoples. Much of the Western Hemisphere was depopulated by diseases, with none causing more deaths than smallpox. While population density, genetics, and the newness of the illnesses all played a role in the destruction wrought by pestilence in the New World, so too did the various medical beliefs and practices of those who lived there.

DISEASE TREATMENT IN PRE-COLUMBIAN AMERICA

The medical beliefs of the different Native American cultures and the varied practices they used to combat illness all bore resemblances to those of other early cultures around the world. Apart from a reliance on prayer and exorcism, the use of medicinal plants and other local agents was common. Tribes stretching from the Great Plains to Central America also utilized sweat lodges to combat illness. Referred to as *temazcal* by the Aztec, *inipi* by the Sioux, and *zumpul-che* by the Maya, these structures were designed to help sweat the disease out of an individual. Unfortunately, dehydration was a serious danger of the practice. For those already suffering from such diuretic diseases as cholera or yellow fever, the cure would merely have worsened the patient's condition. Following the time spent in the sweat lodge, many cultures plunged the individual into cold water, a practice that could produce shock or heart failure in an already weakened patient.[12] Likewise, though Cortés reported advanced apothecaries within the Aztec capital, their overreliance on bleeding as a form of personal sacrifice undoubtedly presented an easy invasion route for disease into the empire.

Various other methods employed by the tribes of the New World included ceremonial dances and prayer ceremonies around the victim. The close contact required for such events would have helped to spread communicable diseases. Some tribes focused on fasting or emetics, which further weaken both the healthy and the infected.[13] Álvar Núñez Cabeza de Vaca reported Native priests massaging diseased victims, after which they "make a few cuts where the pain is located and then suck the skin around the incisions . . . they then breathe on the spot where the pain is and believe that with this the disease goes away."[14]

In addition, the early Spanish and English settlers reported no attempts at practicing quarantine by Indigenous peoples. On the contrary, village members crowded into the homes of the infected to perform ceremonies or care for the sick. Roger Williams reported such a practice among the Native peoples of Rhode Island, writing that when a person was sick, his friends and family crowded around him, "like a quire [*sic*] in prayer to their God for them."[15] Once death did take place, burial practices by some cultures proved equally advantageous to the spread of disease. Thomas Harriot recorded in his *A Brief and True Report of the New Found Land of Virginia* how the deceased among the local people had their bodies opened, their flesh removed, and their bones dried. Undoubtedly during a time of epidemic, these types of practices would have contributed to the spread of a disease.

Though largely ineffective, and at worse counterproductive, for the treatment of illness, many of these practices carried on into the colonial period. While some practices were simply continued with little alteration, others were modified and adopted into Spanish medical practices and Catholic worship as part of the syncretism that dominated the combination of cultures in the sixteenth and seventeenth centuries. These dueling traditions challenged Balmis's efforts and those of his fellow physicians in the early 1800s.

DISEASE AND ITS TREATMENT IN NEW SPAIN

Smallpox first appeared in the New World in 1507, only a decade and a half after the arrival of Columbus. The disease made landfall on the island of Hispaniola, most likely carried by a Spanish sailor. While its impact on the small European population of the island was negligible, its effects on the Natives of the island were apparently catastrophic. August Hirsch later wrote that "whole tribes were exterminated by it."[16] Because of the limited nature of Spanish contacts with the American continent at the time, the disease remained largely confined to the Caribbean islands. The illness seems to have then burned itself out and disappeared from the West.

The Taíno people were decimated by several subsequent outbreaks of the disease, however, beginning with the permanent arrival of the illness in 1517. While Hirsch and others have argued for an African origin of the illness, arriving with enslaved people brought to the Caribbean, smallpox was also reported present in Spain around the same time. With enslaved people being legally imported into the region each year and thousands more illegally brought in, contrary to quotas set by the Spanish crown, it is tempting to connect this mass movement of humans with the spread of the much deadlier variola major, though the evidence for this is insufficient. Regardless of the virus's origin, the epidemic appears to have killed off at least one-third of the Indigenous population of the island of Hispaniola.[17] From there, it quickly spread through trade and with refugees to other islands of the West Indies, killing hundreds of thousands, including half the population of Puerto Rico.[18] This was the same outbreak of the illness that Pánfilo de Narváez brought to Yucatán and transmitted to Cortés's army and, eventually, to Tenochtitlán. The new disease did not stop at the Aztec capital but spread throughout the empire in central Mexico and presumably along the trade routes leading north and south. Only the geography of the border regions of Mesoamerica and the rapidly thinning population densities of surrounding tribal areas served to halt the spread of the epidemic.

Much as in Europe, further waves of the disease began to periodically appear and wash over the populations of the New World, eventually reaching the distant shores of the continents. The Spanish recorded epidemics in various parts of South America in 1533, 1535, 1554, 1566, 1580, 1585, 1588, and 1586–90. The last of these was particularly deadly, with contemporaneous sources claiming it killed off nearly 90 percent of the native population of modern-day Colombia.[19] "They died by scores and hundreds. Villages were depopulated. Corpses were scattered over the fields or piled up in the houses or huts."[20] By the middle part of the century, Chile had been reached by the disease as well, where the virus once again devastated the local population.

Interestingly, it was the French who brought the virus to Brazil. Landing in 1555, a group of Huguenots seeking to escape the religious persecution and death awaiting them back home brought with them not only a new religion but also smallpox, which proceeded to annihilate the Indigenous peoples of the southern Atlantic coast. A decade later, a 1562 epidemic brought by the Portuguese to the region of Bahia is said to have killed off nearly thirty thousand people in only three months.[21] Spanish and Portuguese efforts to concentrate the Indigenous population into plantations, mining colonies, encomiendas, and Jesuit reductions (mission towns) increased the susceptibility of Native peoples to epidemics. In fact, disease emerged as one of the prime reasons for the failure and abandonment of the Jesuit missions in the Marinas region of South America, an area covering much of Peru and the Amazon jungle.[22]

Apart from its effects on human health, the disease also affected the economy of the early Spanish colonies. The decimation of local tribes from smallpox when combined with the meager influx of Spanish immigrants led landowners to rely more heavily on forced labor by enslaved people. The view that Africans were resilient to the malaria that hampered European efforts to colonize the sugar-rich islands of the Caribbean led to an increased trade in humans between the Old and New Worlds. But enslaved Africans were not immune to the outbreaks of epidemic disease. Hemorrhagic smallpox, which emerged in Maranhão (São Luís) in 1660, is said to have killed forty-four thousand persons. An additional deadly eruption of variola major in Brazil in 1665 devastated both Europeans and Africans. Originating in Pernambuco before heading south to Rio de Janeiro, the illness decimated the enslaved people there. A reappearance of the disease in 1669 killed an additional twenty-two thousand, further reducing the population of the colony. The decline in laborers led to a shortage in food being grown and a subsequent famine that affected Brazil well into the 1700s. Portugal's hope for a profitable transatlantic empire was limited by viral and bacterial agents.

Interestingly, while disease was decimating the populations and economies of the various Spanish viceroyalties and Portuguese Brazil, it also prevented several English invasions of the region. In contrast to the effect of disease on the attempts of the Spanish Armada to assault the British Isles, yellow fever and smallpox helped to preserve the Caribbean for Madrid. Notable was an epidemic of yellow fever that swept the area in the 1740s during the War of Jenkins's Ear. Originating in Santo Domingo, the fever moved across the Caribbean in 1740 before being reported as far south as Guayaquil, in modern-day Ecuador. Over the next three years, thousands perished from the illness, with many times that number stricken by it. It was in the midst of this plague that the British attempted to attack the port city of Cartagena de Indias in 1741. The massive expedition, which was composed of over two hundred ships and thirty thousand soldiers and sailors, was almost immediately stricken by disease after its departure. While sickness at sea was something all military commanders at the time prepared for, the death of the expedition's leader, Lord Charles Cathcart, threw the mission into confusion. Worse yet, a major outbreak of typhus the year before had already ravaged half of the Royal Navy's strength.[23]

Even before the assault on the city began, over 500 men had died and 1,500 were confined to their bunks. So many men had been lost that one-third of the soldiers had to be mustered to replace the dead and dying sailors just to allow the fleet to complete its voyage.[24] When the assault on Cartagena and its surrounding forts finally began, losses to disease continued to outpace those from battle. In fact, the Spanish commander Don Blas de Lezo largely relied on delay and disease to protect him from the English, knowing that the sickness season would soon be on them. The initial attack on the Boca Chica forts cost the English 120 killed and wounded, though during the same period they lost 250 from tropical disease, and 600 more were confined to hospitals. By the start of May, Thomas Wentworth could count only 3,200 men as being fit for duty, a number that fell to 1,700 a week later. After it became clear to Wentworth and Edward Vernon that they could not take the city, they withdrew to England, a voyage that cost another 1,100 lives. A final assault by Admiral Vernon aimed at Santiago de Cuba fared little better. Around 4,000 men besieged the city for four months, from July to December of 1741. Various diseases began to infect the army, killing off 2,260 by the end of the year. In all, the expedition lasted for 67 days and saw the deaths of 18,000 men, mostly from disease. The English ultimately withdrew, and both Vernon's career and the War of Jenkins's Ear were over.

Disease dictated the political future of the Caribbean again in the 1760s when another British invasion was met by an outbreak of yellow fever. Following an outbreak at Veracruz in 1761, the illness transited the Caribbean Sea to Cuba. The Havana yellow fever epidemic of 1762 sent thousands of the local Spanish soldiers to the hospital or their graves, severely weakening the island's defenses. A large English invasion force landed in June as part of the campaigns of the Seven Years' War and soon besieged the capital. Though the Spanish governor Juan de Prado hoped to follow de Lezo's example and wait for disease to destroy the British, his own forces were far too enervated to outlast General George Keppel, third Earl of Albemarle. By August 13, Havana had fallen. Yet, as was typical of the various wars of the century, the island's seizure was only temporary, and Cuba was exchanged once more during treaty negotiations. Despite this, the British lost an estimated fifteen thousand men to illness during their yearlong occupation. Continuing the tragedy, returning British and American soldiers transmitted yellow fever back to Philadelphia in 1741 and 1763.

Epidemic disease remained a danger for the Spanish colonists as well. One of the most serious outbreaks occurred from 1736 to 1737. Referred to a decade later by the local historian Cayetano Cabrera Quintero as an outbreak of matlazahuatl, the exact nature of the pestilence remains debated. Historians and scientists have proposed plague, *Salmonella typhi*, or some unknown hemorrhagic fever as possible causes of the disease. According to Quintero, the disease originated in a textile shop in Tacuba, in Mexico City, in November of 1736, and by the turn of the new year it had spread throughout the Valley of Mexico. Tens of thousands were sickened, with Cabrera reporting over forty thousand deaths in Mexico City alone. In response, the city council ordered over a dozen religious processions and novenaries, seeking divine intervention to help assuage the onslaught. In addition, they set about cleaning public streets, prohibited the transport of the dead, and lent financial assistance to local hospitals. While the deadly outbreak eventually subsided, it did affect the public health landscape in the region immensely, establishing precedent for future efforts to tackle illness. The traditional alliance of church and state in battling disease was strengthened as well. In fact, claims that the Virgin of Guadalupe had helped to stay the pestilence led to a renewed push for her official adoption as the patroness of the nation.[25] A papal bull issued in 1754, over 220 years after Mary's initial appearance, finally allowed for this. Likewise, civic authorities in New Spain began to take a more active role in helping to organize responses to the outbreak of illness in the viceroyalty.

An outbreak of smallpox in 1776 in Socorro, New Granada (Colombia), quickly turned into an epidemiological disaster as well. Around six thousand of the city's thirty-three thousand residents, a staggering percentage, ultimately died of the disease. As the illness intensified, the poor proved unable to afford burials, and increasing numbers of bodies were soon abandoned in the streets or on the steps of local churches.[26] When combined with the new and intrusive tax policies of the Bourbon reforms, the smallpox epidemic helped to spread the popular unrest that led to the Comunero Rebellion that occurred in the city in 1781.

Though the revolt was quickly put down and little was done to curtail the more unpopular elements of the Bourbon reforms, Madrid did provide for the variolation of local communities in the region in the 1780s. The practice, which most likely originated in China during the twelfth to sixteenth centuries, found its way to the Ottoman Empire, and from there it was brought back to England by Lady Mary Wortley Montagu. As the wife of the English ambassador to the court of the sultan, she became familiar with the process and had her five-year-old son variolated in 1718. Montagu's personal support for the practice brought it to the attention of the future Queen Caroline of England, who had several prisoners variolated before attempting the practice on her own children.

The procedure involved infecting a healthy person with material from the smallpox sores of a person with a mild form of the disease. The newly infected person experiences a less dangerous illness and develops immunity from the disease. The practice spread throughout much of Europe and is first reported in Spain in 1728.[27] Despite this early appearance, the country seems to have been slow in undertaking the practice on a large scale. Debate over its necessity, its efficacy, and the dangers associated with it delayed its adoption in most nations, particularly in Germany, France, and Spain. Even in New England, Puritan resistance to the procedure turned violent as citizens attempted to murder Cotton Mather, a local supporter of the concept. One English writer who was opposed to the practice praised the Spanish for not following suit: "Spain, which is so much behind the rest of Europe in all mental acquirements, benefited on this occasion by their sluggishness . . . and no other country in Europe has suffered so little from the Small Pox."[28] Many people in Spain, however, were very interested in the practice. In 1772, the twenty-three-year-old Dr. Miguel O'Gorman, who later helped to introduce inoculation to Buenos Aires and opened the first medical school in the region of Argentina, traveled to London to learn the process and upon his return used it on several noble patients.

The use of the practice in the New World seems to have been tied to economic concerns and fears of public safety rather than to purely humanitarian aims. French plantation owners on Saint-Domingue began to utilize variolation as early as 1745. With the annual arrival of slave ships, inoculation was essential to prevent epidemics that could produce possible economic collapse. In 1767, M. de la Chapelle performed a mass inoculation of his entire plantation, a first on the island. Though the practice never became universal in the Caribbean region, many seized on it out of economic necessity.[29] Perhaps hearing of its success on these neighboring islands, authorities in Mexico City began to actively push for the practice in 1779, publishing a work by Dr. Esteban Morel on the subject, in the midst of a major outbreak of the illness.

The call for variolation in various parts of Latin America, in keeping with other regions, was pushed by such factors as economic necessity and fear of political reprisal. Traditional Catholic notions of a duty to care for the sick as well as emerging Enlightenment notions of the proper role of government were also at play. The health of the nation was evolving into a concern for governments. The subsequent development of Edward Jenner's preventative treatment would likewise find its champion among these rulers and elites. Overall, the reasons behind the eventual launching of the Balmis Expedition were multifaceted, being heavily influenced by divergent streams of thought and built on several centuries of devastating experiences with disease in both Spain and its colonies.

CHAPTER 3

The Enlightenment and Disease

It is the business of legislators to watch over the health
of the citizens.

—BARON DE MONTESQUIEU

THE NOTION OF PUBLIC HEALTH being closely intertwined with the proper role of government stretches back to the very birth of society. From the advanced waste disposal systems constructed at Skara Brae in the Orkney Islands around 3000 BC to medieval regulations in Paris over the use of pigs as tools of waste removal, local and national leaders have been prominent in working toward preventing and treating outbreaks of illness. From early religious notions to royal dictates, the responsibility for these developments has paralleled the centralization of power by leaders in recent centuries.

Early humans generally looked toward the supernatural as both the cause of and the solution to their health worries. Disease was viewed by many cultures as a punishment, one to be corrected by appeasing the gods, spirits, or ancestors. Within Chinese epidemiology, specifically, notions of health were closely intertwined with morality and action.

> When the emperor is unjust in reward and punishment and not judicious in hearing lawsuits, Heaven visits him with disease and calamities, and frost and dew will be untimely.[1]

This belief was a cornerstone of the Zhou-era political philosophy of the Mandate of Heaven, which argued that the emperor's right to rule was granted by the gods because of his moral uprightness. Conversely, a lack of morality in a ruler could lead to his justified overthrow. The problem inherent in this right to revolution, however, is in determining whether the ruler has lost his authority. Later Confucian scholars, most notably Dong Zhongshu, argued that the appearance of terrible portents, including famine, flood, and disease, would reveal an emperor's loss of the Mandate of Heaven. Therefore, various Chinese emperors not only took extraordinary steps to ensure their own health and longevity but also actively worked to ameliorate epidemics. Parallels of this can also be found in the Western tradition. Oedipus's decision to blind himself went beyond the symbolic to reflect a belief in the inability of a deformed or unhealthy monarch practically and legitimately to hold on to power.

In the West, views of illness, whether personal or epidemic, were also heavily influenced by the concept of monotheistic religion. God was at the same time a source of illness and a wellspring of healing. The former role did not imply that all disease was from God, but that He certainly was capable of using it as a form of punishment. As stated in Exodus 15:26, "He said, 'If you listen carefully to the Lord your God and do what is right in his eyes, if you pay attention to his commands and keep all his decrees, I will not bring on you any of the diseases I brought on the Egyptians, for I am the Lord, who heals you.'" The physical and viral plagues that struck the Egyptians were seen by the Jews as a form of divine punishment. Likewise strict adherence to the laws of Judaism were seen as preventing a similar fate for the Israelites. Several centuries later, in 701 BC, an Assyrian assault on Jerusalem was miraculously stopped by an outbreak of pestilence that decimated the besieging army. Lord Byron's "The Destruction of Sennacherib" highlights the divine nature of the illness.

> For the Angel of Death spread his wings on the blast,
> And breathed in the face of the foe as he passed;
> And the eyes of the sleepers waxed deadly and chill,
> And their hearts but once heaved—and for ever grew still!

Jewish history is full of God using illness as a weapon against the enemies of Israel.

Building on these ideas, Mosaic code concerned itself with the spiritual health of the Jews as well as their physical well-being. Prohibitions on the consumption of certain animals and food products have been read by some as being as much about health as a test of religious devotion. Rules established within the religion concerning childbirth and circumcision were also quite advanced in medical thinking. "If a woman has conceived, and borne a male child, then she shall be unclean seven days; as in the days of her customary impurity she shall be unclean."[2] The isolation of mother and child and the mandated washing of those coming into contact with them would have dramatically reduced certain causes of child mortality. Even the practice of circumcision, which has been shown to provide some health benefits to the baby, was governed by rules of timing and practice to ensure the health of the infant.

Finally, God was seen as a cure for all illness through His omnipotence. Numerous examples exist in the Bible of individuals praying for relief from personal sickness and being granted it by divine intervention. The Old Testament mentions episodes of epidemic illness averted through a similar manner. Two of the more famous episodes of this involve Aaron and David. In the former instance, Aaron used prayer and incense to stop a plague that allegedly killed 14,700 Israelites: "And Aaron took as Moses commanded, and ran into the midst of the congregation; and, behold, the plague was begun among the people: and he put on incense, and made an atonement for the people. And he stood between the dead and the living; and the plague was stayed."[3] Likewise, David's own transgressions brought disease again onto Israel.

So the Lord sent a plague on Israel from that morning until the end of the time designated, and seventy thousand of the people from Dan to Beersheba died. When the angel stretched out his hand to destroy Jerusalem, the Lord relented concerning the disaster and said to the angel who was afflicting the people, "Enough! Withdraw your hand." The angel of the Lord was then at the threshing floor of Araunah the Jebusite. When David saw the angel who was striking down the people, he said to the Lord, "I have sinned; I, the shepherd, have done wrong. These are but sheep. What have they done? Let your hand fall on me and my family.[4]

These beliefs are closely paralleled in the New Testament, where Jesus heals a number of sick and injured people. Following his crucifixion, the power of healing was passed on to his apostles.

And these signs will accompany those who believe: In my name they will drive out demons; they will speak in new tongues; they will pick up snakes with their hands; and when they drink deadly poison, it will not hurt them at all; they will place their hands on sick people, and they will get well.[5]

This was exemplified by Peter's healing of the lame beggar in Acts 3:1–10: "Then Peter said, 'Silver or gold I do not have, but what I do have I give you. In the name of Jesus Christ of Nazareth, walk.' Taking him by the right hand, he helped him up, and instantly the man's feet and ankles became strong. He jumped to his feet and began to walk."[6]

With the decline of civic institutions in Western Europe following the collapse of Rome, the Church took over many of the functions of the state. Most notable among these was the handling of the sick and injured. In contrast with the Protestant nations of Europe, the Catholic Church remained heavily involved in the process of disease treatment well into the modern era. It was a role that the Catholic Church had participated in since its founding. Jesus's command to his followers, "Heal the sick, raise the dead, cleanse lepers, cast out demons. You received without paying; give without pay," made traditional notions of familial and community responsibility for the caregiving of those afflicted with illness a general religious duty.[7] With the rise of monasteries in the early medieval period, monks and nuns took on the task of spiritually and physically caring for those around them. The sixth-century *Rule of St. Benedict* directly states the following:

Before and above all things, care must be taken of the sick, that they be served in very truth as Christ is served; because He hath said, 'I was sick and you visited Me' (Mt 25:36). And 'As long as you did it to one of these My least brethren, you did it to Me' (Mt 25:40). But let the sick themselves also consider that they are served for the honor of God, and let them not grieve their brethren who serve them by unnecessary demands. These must, however, be patiently borne with, because from such as these a more bountiful reward is gained. Let the Abbot's greatest concern, therefore, be that they suffer no neglect.

Let a cell be set apart for the sick brethren, and a God-fearing, diligent, and careful attendant be appointed to serve them. Let the use of the bath be offered to the sick as often as it is useful, but let it be granted more rarely to the healthy and especially the young. Thus also let the use of meat be granted to the sick and to the very weak for their recovery. But when they have been restored let them all abstain from meat in the usual manner.

But let the Abbot exercise the utmost care that the sick are not neglected by the Cellarer or the attendants, because whatever his disciples do amiss falleth back on him.[8]

This general provision calling for the aid of sick monks and nuns soon involved the treatment of the local population as well. Perhaps the first Spanish hospital to be established, built at Mérida around 580, was a xenodochium designed specifically to help diseased travelers and pilgrims. It became seen as a form of religious devotion to care for the sick and poor.

In Spain, specifically, a tradition of Islamic hospitals built to care for the public readily complemented the preexisting monastic care facilities. Thus, by the onset of the sixteenth century, Spanish medical theory and care were at the forefront of Europe. With the establishment of colonies in the New World, this system was soon exported to the Americas as well. In fact, as early as 1503, the governor of Hispaniola commissioned the construction of the first European hospital in the Western Hemisphere. The Hospital San Nicolás de Bari was built in Santo Domingo over the course of twenty years and at its height was large enough to accommodate seventy patients. Hernán Cortés followed suit when he entered Mexico, ordering the construction of a hospital in Tenochtitlán in 1524 that would eventually become the Hospital de Jesús Nazareno. Throughout the sixteenth and seventeenth centuries, additional church-run hospitals and small missions were established across the Spanish colonies. In contrast, the first public hospital in the English colonies was not built until 1751, when it was established in Philadelphia by Benjamin Franklin and Thomas Bond.

Old religious notions of caring for the poor and infirm meshed well with the colonial caste system that developed in the region. In the colonies in the Americas, this manifested as a care for the Indigenous groups living under Spanish suzerainty. While most hospitals focused on time-tested European methods, the Jesuits, with their usual penchant for combining traditional methods with local customs, welcomed Native American practices. During an outbreak of smallpox in Brazil in the seventeenth century, priests employed medicine, leeches, washing, and prayer, while Indigenous healers are reported to have tried placing victims on stick beds over smoking fires to fumigate the disease. Despite this, the Catholic Church remained at the forefront of medical care throughout much of the colonial time period. Jesuit priests, especially, helped to push attempts at variolation, conducting such operations in the Amazon region as early as the 1720s.[9]

At the same time, the construction of public hospitals represented an attempt by medieval monarchs to shift power away from the Church and toward themselves. In keeping with this trend, several medieval kings began to claim the ability to cure illness, chief among which was scrofula. Tuberculous cervical lymphadenitis, better known as the king's evil, involved a growing chronic mass on the neck, making the disease one of the more visible illnesses of the Middle Ages. Future kings and queens would use the practice of curing through touch not only to legitimize their position but also to demonstrate their divine right to rule. William of Malmesbury wrote,

> But now to speak of his miracles. A young woman had married a husband of her own age, but having no issue by the union, the humours collecting abundantly about her neck, she had contracted a sore disorder; the glands swelling in a dreadful manner. Admonished in a dream to have the part affected washed by the king, she entered the palace, and the king himself fulfilled this labour of love, by rubbing the woman's neck with his fingers dipped in water. Joyous health followed his healing hand: the lurid skin opened, so that worms flowed out with the purulent matter, and the tumour subsided. But as the orifice of the ulcers was large and unsightly, he commanded her to be supported at the royal expense till she should be perfectly cured. However, before a week was expired, a fair, new skin returned, and hid the scars so completely, that nothing of the original wound could be discovered: and within a year becoming the mother of twins, she increased the admiration of Edward's holiness. Those who knew him more intimately, affirm that he often cured this complaint in Normandy.[10]

Debate exists as to whether the practice of the king's touch first began in England with Edward the Confessor or in France with Philip I, both of whom reigned in the eleventh century. Regardless, much as with the contemporaneous Investiture Controversy, such practices presented an opportunity for the monarchy to strip power away from the Church.

Interestingly, the king's touch seems not to have risen as a belief in medieval Spain. The most popular story there concerning a monarch's efforts to heal a sick subject revolves around faith and prayer. Alfonso X of Castile, who reigned from 1252 to 1284, is said to have been approached by a mother seeking a cure for her daughter. According to the *Cantigas de Santa María*, number 321, the girl had been stricken with an inflammation in her neck, possibly scrofula, for several years. A stranger said to her mother,

Good woman, may our Lord help me,
all Christian kings have the power to heal this
malady merely by placing their hands on it.[11]

Rather than perform the miracle, Alfonso X strongly rebuked the parents: "When you say I have this power, you are speaking nonsense."[12] Instead, the Castilian monarch commanded them to pray to the Virgin Mary for succor, and after several days of devotion the girl was cured. This particular cantiga opens with the general axiom:

"O que mui tarde ou nunca, se póde por meezinna,
sãar, en mui pouco tempo, guareç' a Santa Reínna.

(What is often late or never occurs, it is possible for me to do
in a very short time, through the protection of the Holy Queen.)

Alfonso X, also known as Alfonso the Wise, saw the proper role of the king to be that of directing his sickly subjects toward the Church for healing.

Though medieval Spanish kings were clearly aware of the professed power of various other Western European monarchs, the actions of Alfonso X demonstrate that they preferred their subjects to rely on divine intervention instead. But two centuries of marriage alliances with England and France eventually altered the Spanish perception of the throne's power.[13] By the time of Alfonso XI's coronation in 1312, mention is made of the fact that "kings receive such power that they live in God's service and work miracles during their lives of the so-called malady of kings." Despite this proclamation, no reference is ever given of Alfonso XI, or of any other monarch, in fact practicing the feat. Disease management in Spain remained largely driven by a combination of practical science and devout religious observation.

The rise of Protestantism complemented the centuries-old efforts of European monarchs to move authority away from the Church and toward the throne. The dissolution of monasteries and nunneries in England created a unique public health dilemma as there were little to no civic institutions capable of replacing them. Some existing hospitals, such as St. Bartholomew's in London and Charterhouse in Hull, were placed under municipal control, while others, such as the Hospital of St. Lawrence in Acton, were turned into grand homes for loyal followers of the monarch. Though a general decline in the treatment of disease most likely occurred in England and Central Europe during the sixteenth century, monarchs soon exerted their power and filled the vacuum left by the Church. What was formerly a religious duty, providing aid and comfort to the ill, soon became a mark of political power. In this, the kings and queens of Europe were driven by political and epidemiological necessity as well as by the new philosophies of the Enlightenment.

Debates over the proper role and power of government that characterized the Enlightenment included discussions on the notions of public health. Thomas Hobbes, while not directly referencing the role of the ruler in this field, did frequently use the metaphor of disease to address the issues of civil society. Specifically in chapter 29 of the *Leviathan*, Hobbes posits that "though nothing can be immortal which mortals make; yet, if men had the use of reason they pretend to, their Commonwealths might be secured, at least, from perishing by internal diseases."[14] Over the course of the subsequent chapter, he compares the various causes of the dissolution of commonwealths to well-known diseases of the body and mind. While Hobbes falls short of recommending that the king was responsible for the health of the nation, his assertion that it was the monarch's duty to protect the natural rights of his subjects seems to include it as a possible power.

Sir Thomas More's *Utopia* pushes Hobbes's argument to this extreme by detailing the construction of publicly funded and run hospitals in his perfect country.

But they take more care of their sick than of any others; these are lodged and provided for in public hospitals. They have belonging to every town four hospitals, that are built without their walls, and are so large that they may pass for little towns; by this means, if they had ever such a number of sick persons, they could lodge them conveniently, and at such a distance that such of them as are sick of infectious diseases may be kept so far from the rest that there can be no danger of contagion. The hospitals are furnished and stored with all things that are convenient for the ease and recovery of the sick; and those that are put in them are looked after with such tender and watchful care, and are so constantly attended by their skillful physicians, that as none is sent to them against their will, so there is scarce one in a whole town that, if he should fall ill, would not choose rather to go thither than lie sick at home.[15]

Montesquieu, in his *The Spirit of Laws*, deals specifically with the power of government to address disease. After detailing the arrival of leprosy in Western Europe, he points to the actions of King Rothari of the Lombards in not only expelling a leper from the land but making him "incapable of disposing of his property; because from the very moment he had been turned out of his house he was reckoned dead in the eye of the law. In order to prevent all communication with lepers, they were rendered incapable of civil acts."[16] The philosopher then comments on the arrival of syphilis from the New World and states that "as it is the business of legislators to watch over the health of the citizens, it would have been a wise part in them to have stopped this communication by laws made on the plan of those of Moses."[17] Interestingly, Montesquieu cautions against the construction of large numbers of public hospitals that also provided charity services, fearing that "all the hospitals in the world cannot cure this private poverty; on the contrary, the spirit of indolence, which it constantly inspires, increases the general, and consequently the private, misery."[18] While the ruler should address the health issues of the nation as a whole, an excessive focus on the health of the individual would lead to laziness and dependency.

Both the Renaissance and the Enlightenment exposed European rulers and thinkers to greater parts of history and the larger world. It was soon discovered that disease was a universal feature of civilization, not merely a localized element. This concept began to chip away at the traditional views of personal disease management as well as the miasma theory. If disease was universal, then it needed a universal, organized response.

The hope of the Enlightenment, to move man away from superstition and religion and toward reason, coincided with the growth of science, particularly in the field of medicine. Despite the belief in *la polémica de la ciencia española* that became popular following the publication in 1782 of Nicolas Masson de Morvilliers's work that lamented the lack of scientific advancement in Spain with such prejudicial statements as, "Spain, which is so much behind the rest of Europe in all mental acquirements," the nation had been at the forefront of medical innovation in the sixteenth century.[19] Some of these innovations resulted from the strong foundations established by the various thinkers of the Caliphate of Córdoba. While Europe was just emerging from the Middle Ages, the Islamic region of the Iberian Peninsula was importing knowledge from the Middle East as well reaching new heights in science and medicine on its own. Such legendary scientists and doctors as Ḥisdai ibn Shaprut, Ibn Juljul, Abū al-Qāsim al-Zahrāwī, and Ibn Zuhr made Córdoba the forefront of medical knowledge in the Western world. Geoffrey Chaucer even made reference to "Olde Ypocras [Hippocrates], Haly and Galeyn [Galen], Serapion, Razi [Rhazes] and Avycen [Avicenna]" as famed doctors in the prologue to his *The Canterbury Tales*. At the same time, state-sponsored hospitals were constructed throughout Al-Andalus, most of which continued their operations following the Reconquista. Spanish respect for the connection between royal and national health was seen when the nobility removed Sancho the Fat of Leon, who reigned from 959 to 966, from power in part because of his ill-health and obesity. 'Abd al-Raḥmān III of Córdoba agreed to aid in his restoration and also sent his personal physician, Hasdai ibn Shaprut, to treat his condition.

The influence of Islamic learning can be clearly seen in the accomplishments of perhaps the greatest Spanish scientist of the medieval period, Arnold of Villanova. The thirteenth-century scholar and doctor understood Arabic and was able to directly access works produced in Córdoba.

He taught at the medical school at Montpellier, is credited with treating three popes, and wrote over one hundred works. He perfected the method of extracting essential oils from plants and herbs with alcohol and recommended wine as both a therapeutic substance and an antiseptic: "If wine is taken in right measure it suits every age, every time, and every region."[20]

Spain's territorial advances in the sixteenth century were likewise complemented by developments in science. A Siglo de Oro in the fields of medicine and invention characterized much of the century. Some of the great thinkers of the period included Andrés Alcázar, who pioneered surgical techniques; Francisco Díaz de Alcalá, who founded urology; Bartolomé Hidalgo de Agüero, who introduced the dry healing of stab wounds; Miguel Servet, who first described pulmonary circulation; and Francisco Valles, who focused on medicinal plants. Juan Tomás Porcell, who lived from 1528 to 1580, wrote perhaps the first epidemiological treatise on bubonic plague. Following an outbreak of the disease in Zaragoza in 1564, Porcell gathered statistical and anatomical data on all sufferers, combining the information into a manuscript the next year. Likewise, Juan de Villarreal and Luis Mercado wrote extensively in 1611 and 1613, respectively, on the symptoms and treatment of diphtheria.

Alongside many Spanish advancements in medicine, the Enlightenment was also present on Spanish soil. In fact, much of the origin of Enlightenment thought can be traced to ideas developed in the School of Salamanca in the sixteenth century. Francisco de Vitoria's teachings on international law and just war theory, Domingo de Soto's writings on usury and banking, Martín de Azpilcueta and Tomás de Mercado's work on monetary theory, and Francisco Suárez's work on natural rights and natural law preceded other Enlightenment thinkers by a century. The culmination of this movement can be seen in the works of Friar Benito Jerónimo Feijóo y Montenegro, whose early eighteenth-century works pushed for the scientific method, combated superstition, and argued for improvements in medicine and public health efforts. Though a strong devotion to Catholicism remained a dominant feature in Spanish thought, other elements associated with the Enlightenment were readily adopted by the kingdoms of the region.

Absolutism, however, arrived late in the Iberian Peninsula. Spain had a long history of establishing apparatuses to limit the power of the monarch, with some arguing that the roots of these lay in the various councils of Toledo that dominated the Visigothic kingdom.[21] In fact, the first establishment of a permanent parliament in Continental Europe occurred in León, years before similar bodies arose in England or France. In 1188, the embattled Alfonso IX called together his Curia Regis and representatives of the towns and cities of his kingdom for advice and legislative action. Over the next century, similar assemblies were held in Castile and Aragon. Though the Cortes of León and Castile gradually became combined, after the unification of those territories by Ferdinand III (Saint Ferdinand) in the thirteenth century, the Cortes of Castile and Aragon remained separate even after the unification of Spain. These parliamentary bodies served to limit the powers of the monarchy. With the general decline of royal authority during the late seventeenth century because of medical issues, especially during the reign of Charles II, power in Spain appeared to be shifting more toward the parliaments. This stood in contrast with what was occurring in the various other states of Europe at the time. Had it not been for the outcome of the War of the Spanish Succession, the degeneration and demise of the house of Habsburg in Spain could have seen the birth of a constitutional monarchy years before it occurred in England.

The arrival of the House of Bourbon in Spain in 1700 under the personage of Philip V altered this trajectory. The French royal brought with him a much more centralized concept of rule, reminiscent of his grandfather, Louis XIV. The new king promulgated the Nueva Planta decrees, which effectively unified the diverse legislative and advisory councils within Spain. The various regional Cortes that had existed for almost seven hundred years were now united. At the same time, the charters, grants, and privileges that were present in the kingdoms and provinces, such as the Catalan constitutions and Furs of Valencia, were stripped away or standardized. The Bourbon reforms sought to insert the monarchy into the social, religious, and economic problems of the nation in an effort to modernize the country.

Though initial efforts undertaken during Philip V's reign, under the guidance of Cardinal Giulio Alberoni, did seek to address issues arising in the colonies, their dominant focus on securing and expanding Spanish power in Europe through military means severely limited their success overseas. Only with the rise of Ferdinand VI and his chief minister Zenón de Somodevilla y Bengoechea, marquis de la Ensenada, did the Bourbon reforms begin to focus more on the well-being of the Spanish Empire. As one historian noted, "The new regime accepted that Spain's interest resided not in European battlefields but in the Atlantic and beyond."[22] These efforts proved short lived as Ensenada and, later, José de Carvajal y Lancáster fell from favor, and Ferdinand's wife moved to blunt the reforms. Her sudden death in 1754 sent the king into a severe depression from which he never recovered.

The ascension of Charles III in 1759 seemed to spark an interest once again in aiding and reforming the colonial empire. The temporary loss of Havana to England in 1762 showed the inherent military weakness of the kingdom and further exposed its overreliance on trade with the New World. Charles III subsequently sought to combine the reform agendas of both previous monarchs, focusing on military growth and internal economic improvement. Seeing himself in the guise of an enlightened absolutist, the king sought to strengthen the throne's power to improve the *felicidad publica* of the nation while weakening the traditional power of the various regions and the Church.[23] As the central idea of the Enlightenment revolved around rule by reason, part of Charles III's reforms involved dispatching royal inspectors and intendants to observe the various colonial administrations and ensure the proper working of the colonies. To further aid in economically exploiting these lands to bolster social and military advancement back in Iberia, various scientific expeditions were sent out under royal authority, all of which served as precursors to the Balmis Expedition.

Despite English thinking, Spain and its colonies were hardly the medically, scientifically, and politically backward regions they are often portrayed to be. As has been seen, traditional church practices and Islamic developments served to produce a nation quite advanced in terms of public health care. In the colonies, hospitals were established in New Spain over 250 years before they appeared in New England. The *Mercurio Volante*, arguably the first medical journal of the New World, was published in Mexico in 1772. Arguments over variolation occurred in Madrid at the same time they occurred in London, and the practice became as popular in the former as it was in the latter. Finally, many of the ideas of the Enlightenment can be said to have had their roots in the Iberian Peninsula, especially in the thinking of the School of Salamanca. If anything came belatedly to Spain, it was the notion of absolutism, with its associated negative implications.

CHAPTER 4

Spanish Expeditions of the Eighteenth Century

*I believe that there are many herbs and many trees that
are worth much in Europe for dyes and for medicines.*

—CHRISTOPHER COLUMBUS

THE NECESSITY OF MAXIMIZING preexisting sources of profit from the New World as well as discovering new products pushed the Spanish crown to send a series of scientific expeditions to the Western Hemisphere. Perhaps with its long history of utilizing small bands of conquistadors to explore, conquer, and transform the various Islamic lands of Spain, the nation was accustomed to such undertakings. While expeditions to the New World in the fifteenth and sixteenth centuries were largely exploratory and military in nature, the expeditions of the eighteenth century were much more scientific in purpose. At the same time, the concerns of the various kings for the economic growth and public happiness of their citizens served as strong motivators for these undertakings, all of which served as models for the launching of Balmis's Philanthropic Expedition.

A precursor to the voyages of Charles III and Charles IV was the Francisco Hernández expedition of the late sixteenth century. Born in Toledo and educated at the University of Salamanca, Hernández served as a doctor at a hospital and a monastery in Guadalupe from 1558 to 1562 and at a hospital in Toledo from 1562 to 1567. During this time, he began work on a Spanish translation of Pliny's *Natural History*, a volume that he would model his own writings on a decade later. Because of his exceptional medical skill, Hernández eventually became chief physician to King Philip II in 1567, a position that allowed him to frequently press the monarch for the chance to explore the New World as a sixteenth-century Pliny. Finally, in 1570, Philip appointed him chief physician of the New World and tasked him with undertaking a scientific expedition there. This was more than simply a royal reward for a loyal counselor. The considerable sum of 60,000 ducats was set aside for the voyage, which would take five years to complete, making it an involved, royally sponsored scientific expedition that would serve as a model for Balmis.[1]

Departing in late 1570 and hailing along the way at the Canary Islands, Santo Domingo, and Cuba, Hernández finally made landfall at Veracruz in February of 1571. His route became a standard model for numerous subsequent expeditions, including Balmis's 234 years later. The expedition included among its sizeable contingent painters and a geographer to help Hernández document and place into context the various plants and animals he discovered. Interestingly, most of the artists employed by the physician were Aztec, as were many of the guides, lending a knowledgeable local component to the undertaking. Hernández himself early on pushed Philip to approve his gathering together of Indigenous people to "show them plants so that they may help me to establish the medical virtues and tell me their experience with them."[2] This early expedition saw a distinctive absence of the scientific standardization and absolutism of later voyages. This voyage was more directed by the beliefs of the Renaissance, which placed value on experience and the lessons of the past.

From early on in his exploration, the royal physician emphasized the medical advantages that could be gained from a proper understanding of the New World's natural environment: "As I understand it, this will be such a grand enterprise that there will be no need to bring to the Indies medicines from Spain, nor to Spain from Alexandria."[3] From 1571 to 1574, Hernández explored the length of Mexico and Central America, describing the natural and medicinal properties of thousands of plants and animals. Some of his more interesting discoveries and descriptions included pineapples, corn, *Guaiacum officinale*, smilax, *Strychnos nux-vomica*, sweet granadilla, passion fruit, peyote, agave, datura, and *Chenopodium*, the last of which Indigenous peoples in the region used as a treatment for dysentery. It is believed that Hernández was one of the first to document the use of chocolate as a drink by the Mexica people. His descriptions of the product, and his own beliefs of its potential usage to cure fevers, sparked a century-long interest in Europe of chocolate as a curative agent.[4]

Hernández quickly realized the broader humanitarian result of his accomplishment, writing to the king in April of 1572: "I understand now that I have finished writing about it . . . that the Indies could provide medicines for the whole world without the need to ship them from any other place at all."[5] The American colonies could both enrich Spain and provide medical help to Europe. To further these ends, Hernández spent much of 1574–77 performing numerous medical experiments in Mexico with the various new plants he had discovered. In keeping with his desire to allow for the dissemination of his discoveries throughout the European continent, he noted to the king that he was writing his books in Latin, "so that this great gift of Your Majesty's may be communicated to all nations because this is the common language."[6]

Hernández's time in Mexico coincided with the previously mentioned outbreak of huey cocoliztli in 1576. Because of his university training and medical expertise, Hernández, at the request of the viceroy, took up residence in the Hospital Real de Naturales. He examined patients stricken with the illness and kept careful observations of its spread. Along with several assistants, he also performed autopsies of the bodies of those who fell victim to the pestilence. Hernández's observations remain some of the few descriptions of a mysterious illness that for years was assumed to simply have been smallpox.

After returning to Spain, Dr. Hernández had his works compiled into a massive tome and presented to Philip II. From these, the king commissioned Nardo Antonio Recchi to produce a condensed version in the 1580s, but it would take until 1651 for Recchi's work to be published for an international audience. The praise heaped on the volume was substantial, and a later republishing of it in 1790 most likely served as further inspiration for the launching of the Balmis Expedition.

The late eighteenth century saw the dispatching of several notable scientific expeditions to the Spanish colonies in America. As previously mentioned, Charles III viewed such undertakings as a means by which to satisfy the economic, strategic, medicinal, and social concerns of Spain. From 1777 to 1789, he commissioned five major undertakings that reached both the Americas and Asia. Expanding on the more practical reasons for launching such attempts, his decision to send so many exploratory voyages was also in keeping with his own Enlightenment and absolutist tendencies.

The first of these trips was organized in 1777 and was chiefly a botanical expedition to Peru and Chile. Charles III had been told of the possibility of medicinal plants existing along the western coast of South America that would produce both social and economic returns for his empire.[7] Hipólito Ruiz López and José Antonio Pavón, both of whom were only twenty-three years old and students at the time, were selected to undertake the eleven-year expedition. In their company was the French botanist Joseph Dombey and the artists José Brunete and Isidore Gálvez.[8] Departing from Cádiz in November of 1777, the group made landfall in Lima in April of 1778. Over the next six years, the group traveled throughout the Viceroyalty of Peru collecting and documenting thousands of specimens. While in the city of Concepción in 1782, an outbreak of illness, anachronistically described as cholera, erupted in the region. Dombey's training as a physician made him invaluable in treating the sick and preventing a larger disaster. Much as with the Hernández expedition, Spain gained the materials of the New World, while the colonies benefited from the medical knowledge of the Old.

Despite the expedition's success in gathering materials and providing medical aid to the region, its efforts to return these goods to Spain proved more challenging. An initial sailing in 1780 was captured by a

British warship. The American Revolution was raging at the time, and Spain had recently allied with the colonial cause, thus making Spanish vessels a legitimate target for England. Dombey, after feuding with both López and Pavón, returned to Spain in 1784, only to have most of his plants impounded by customs, in whose possession they eventually died. A fire that broke out in Macará in 1785 destroyed even more samples. Finally, in 1786, fifty-three crates of plants and materials that were aboard the *San Pedro de Alcantara* were lost when the ship sank off the coast of Portugal. Despite these failures, the expedition did manage to gather around 3,000 plants, create over 2,500 illustrations, and set up an herbarium in Quito in 1808. López and Pavón published their findings from 1798 to 1802.

Concurrent with the López-Pavón expedition, José Celestino Mutis led his own botanical exploration of New Granada. Mutis had been living in New Granada since 1760 and in 1763 and 1764 had proposed a voyage to explore the region, only to have the court reject him both times. In 1783, his proposal was finally approved, in part because of the king's sudden botanical interest as well as Mutis's suggestion of the possibility of growing tea in the region. The Spanish naturalist had written about a shrub called *Symplocos theiformis*, which when brewed could produce a delicate tea. Mutis argued that the drink not only had medicinal properties but could circumvent the China tea trade then enriching the British.[9]

Officially launched in April of 1783, the expedition included the botanists Eloy Valenzuela and Fray Diego García; the geographers Bruno Lardete, Francisco José de Caldas, and José Cambler; and the painters Pablo Antonio García, Francisco Javier Matiz, Anthony Cortez, Vicente Sánchez, Antonio Barrionuevo, Vicente Silva, and Salvador Rizo Blanco. The decades-long undertaking straddled many of the revolutionary wars that erupted in the region. In fact, Salvador Rizo and Francisco de Caldas were killed in 1816 fighting against Spain, and the botanist Francisco Antonio Zea served as vice president of Gran Colombia in 1819. Mutis, though, largely confined his work to the scientific, helping to establish a public art school and an astronomical observatory and writing the *Flora de*

Bogotá using the latest in Linnaean classification systems. The naturalist also took a profound interest in the ants of the region, observing them for years and writing hundreds of pages on their behavior and their impact on the region's economy.[10]

Overall, the expedition lasted from 1783 to 1816, surviving even the death of Mutis himself in 1808. It covered an estimated 8,000 square kilometers of territory, documented 6,000 species, and sent 24,000 dried plants and 5,000 drawings to the Royal Botanic Gardens in Madrid. Mutis's own writings documented at least seven new plant species with medicinal powers. In fact, these royal botanical expeditions did much to examine and transmit information about cinchona bark, a preventive aid and cure for malaria. In the sugar-rich Caribbean islands, this illness proved to be far more debilitating to Spanish society and economics then even smallpox was. Though the antimalarial properties of the bark had been known since at least the 1630s, and it had been employed as a curative agent by Charles II of England and Louis XIV of France, detailed botanical information about the tree itself was lacking.

The third companion expedition of the era was launched in 1787 under the command of Martín Sessé y Lacasta and focused on the Spanish Empire's northern region in the Americas. Organized to explore the flora and fauna of New Spain, the expedition lasted until 1803. As with the other expeditions, many notable members composed Sessé's team. Included among these were the botanist Vicente Cervantes, museum of natural history director José Longinos Martínez, pharmacist Juan Diego del Castillo, and the artist Atanasio Echeverría y Godoy. Also accompanying the expedition was José Mariano Mociño, who was later exiled from Spain because of his support for Joseph Bonaparte.

Beginning around the region of Mexico City, the group collected various plants and specimens, all of which were used to establish the Viceregal Botanical Garden in March of 1788, an event that included a majestic fireworks display.[11] From there, Sessé proceeded toward Acapulco before turning north and exploring Michoacán and Jalisco in 1790. The group split at this point, with Mociño, del Castillo, and Echeverría heading toward Aguascaliente, while Sessé investigated the area around Sinaloa in the north. The success and renown of their work is demonstrated by the fact that in 1828, the Swiss botanist Augustin Pyrame de Candolle named the large genus of stonecrops and succulents that inhabit the region from Mexico to northwestern South America *Echeveria* after the expedition's artist.

Suddenly in 1792, an order from Madrid arrived requiring Sessé to direct his efforts toward Nootka Island. Located off Vancouver Island, the entire region had been claimed as de facto Spanish territory since the fifteenth century. But Madrid's failure to effectively colonize or control the area had invited Russian, British, and American interest. A series of minor and belated expeditions sent by Charles III in the 1770s and 1780s failed to impress London regarding Spain's commitment to the area. A boundary dispute over the region soon erupted between Spain and Great Britain, and Charles hoped to use this voyage both to discern the value of the area and to stake a more valid claim during the ongoing Nootka Convention discussions then taking place.

After finishing this great northern excursion, the expedition returned to Mexico. Over the course of 1793 it again split into two parts, exploring the Mixteca Region, Tabasco, Xalapa, and Guazturo before reuniting at Veracruz. The success of Sessé's efforts was demonstrated by the fact that in 1794 he was allowed to continue and expand his efforts into the Caribbean and Guatemala. Again the group divided, with Sessé sailing toward Cuba and Mociño pushing south toward Central America.

By 1803, the expedition was ordered to return to Spain. Overall, Sessé and his fellow explorers documented thousands of species of plants and animals, including many new genera. Though this particular campaign was directed less toward medical matters, Sessé himself wrote extensively on yellow fever in 1804 after returning to Europe. And del Castillo succumbed to the effects of scurvy in 1793 while exploring Mexico, a not uncommon fate on expeditions at the time.

The various expeditions of Charles III were not confined to the Americas but extended to the far reaches of the Spanish Empire, particularly to the Spanish Philippines. The origins of one such expedition to Asia lay with the work of Juan de Cuéllar, who sailed to the Philippine islands in 1786 of his own accord. A trained botanist working in Seville, Cuéllar was no doubt inspired by the contemporaneous work of López and Pavón. Much like the royally sanctioned expeditions, Cuéllar's work combined a scientific interest in nature with a look toward exploiting profitable resources. His early interest in examining and documenting indigo, black pepper, cotton, coffee, and cinnamon clearly demonstrates this.

It was his work with this last item that soon attracted the interest of Madrid. In 1788 Cuéllar received a royal directive to study the possibility of farming cinnamon and nutmeg in the archipelago.[12] Spanish trade in these items was dwarfed by that of the much larger Dutch plantations in the East Indies. Growing cinnamon in the Philippines could potentially make the islands as profitable as the sugar plantations in the Spanish West Indies.

To discover the possibilities of pursuing this economic venture, a large expedition was fitted out in Spain and sent on a voyage across the Atlantic and Pacific Oceans. The Malaspina Expedition, named after its commander, Alessandro Malaspina, crossed the Atlantic in 1789 and hugged the western coast of the Americas. Composed of two ships, the *Descubierta* and the *Atrevida*, the expedition would eventually dwarf James Cook's accomplishments and discovery of a generation before.[13] The expedition's initial goal was influenced, in part, by strategic concerns. Russian interest in Alaska was increasing, and the Spanish felt obligated once again to demonstrate their interest in the area. While these diplomatic achievements were short lived, Malaspina's scientific discovery in the region proved to be much more important.

After landing near Nootka Sound, Malaspina and his men employed a Native American technique of brewing spruce beer and conifer tea to combat scurvy. Likewise, his ship's surgeon, Pedro González, insisted on

supplying the crew with fresh oranges and lemons. Because of this combination, the expedition saw almost no outbreak of the disease and zero
casualties from it despite circumnavigating the planet, a rarity for the time
period. In comparison, the vast majority of the losses in Vacso de Gama's
and Ferdinand Magellan's voyages were from scurvy, and British attempts
to explore the Pacific in the eighteenth century were plagued by the disease
as well.[14]

In March of 1792, the two Spanish ships finished their crossing of the
Pacific and made landfall at Cavite, in the Philippines, after a rather peace-
ful voyage. Apart from performing general repairs and exploring the area,
Malaspina and his scientists met with Cuéllar and took some of his samples
and drawings aboard. The ships remained in the region until November,
before turning south toward Australia and New Zealand.

These expeditions are all the more interesting for the way in which they
incorporated elements of both the Enlightenment and absolutism, something that would be more fully reflected in the Balmis Expedition. While
the Enlightenment brought about an interest in the systematic study of
nature, its tendency to exclude more traditional methods and focus on the
forceful application of universally accepted methods of inquiry lent itself to
scientific absolutism, and in the case of the New World, scientific imperialism.[15] In Mexico, local Spanish and traditional Nahua names for plants
were shunned for the Latin naming system popularized by Linnaeus. To
aid in this, yearly botanical exercises were held at the garden in Mexico
City. University students undertook a public examination in which they
were required to name various specimens. This process would have been
similar to those employed at similar institutions in Iberia.[16] Local reactions
to this process would have been mixed, with some lamenting the loss of
traditional naming systems and fearing the overreach of Madrid, which
now encroached even into the field of science. While scientific absolutism
could be directed to destroy other modes of investigation and folk ideas,
it was also used to elevate colonial institutions and universities to a level
of parity with Spain. This would have given hope to local Criollos that

perhaps their training and status would be accepted as comparable to that of the Peninsulares.

Overall, Charles III's interest in exploring the natural landscape of his empire rested on several key premises. There clearly was a desire to discover and exploit the economic blessings of the various regions. Mutis's focus on bypassing the tea trade from China, efforts to capitalize on the trade of cinchona, and Dombey's efforts to investigate mining possibilities in Peru and Chile demonstrate this. At the same time, the Enlightenment notions of applying reason to the world around us and investigating for the sake of investigation were also present, as were the absolutist notions of establishing control over the various components, natural and man-made, of the nation. Finally, the thought that the government should strive to support its citizens' health and socioeconomic well-being served as an overarching theme. These were not simply transitory undertakings for Charles III. His commitment of over 300,000 pesos to the various projects shows a dedication to the aforementioned principles, one which would culminate in the launching of the Royal Philanthropic Vaccine Expedition by his son and heir.[17]

CHAPTER 5

Jenner as John the Baptist

I am the voice of one crying out in the desert,
"Make straight the way of the Lord."

—JOHN 1:23

SIR FRANCIS DARWIN, famed botanist and son of the popularizer of the idea of evolution through natural selection, once opined that "in science, credit goes to the man who convinces the world, not the man to whom the idea first occurs."[1] While the quote works well for the fact that Charles Darwin largely popularized rather than developed the hypothesis of evolution, it also describes the life of Sir Edward Jenner. The pioneer of the smallpox vaccination did far more to test and popularize an already suspected notion than to actually create it. His accomplishments were nevertheless revolutionary and necessary for the Balmis Expedition to occur.

Jenner was born in May of 1749 in Berkeley, England. Located in a vale between the Severn River and the Cotswold Edge, this dairy-producing region provided the natural catalysts for Jenner's eventual triumph. As was common in the age, he was apprenticed after turning thirteen, to a local surgeon. Traveling thirty miles to the south, near the city of Bristol, Jenner learned the skill of medicine from a local doctor. According to lore, it was there that Jenner heard a milkmaid exclaim, "I shall never have smallpox for I have had cowpox." Cowpox was a relatively minor illness, typically contracted by milkmaids from infected cattle. As the viruses that caused cowpox and smallpox were within the same genus, the contraction of one would lead to resistance of the other. The veracity of the tale matters less than does the apparently present belief that cowpox protected against smallpox.[2] How widespread the belief was at the time is difficult to gauge, but others in the region had certainly heard the tales as well.

One of these was Benjamin Jesty, who lived from 1737 to 1816. As a farmer in North Dorset, England, Jesty would have almost certainly heard tales about cowpox immunity. In 1774, during an outbreak of smallpox in the area, he put these tales to the test. Jesty used material from an infected cow's udder to vaccinate his wife and two sons, all of whom quickly weathered the resulting cowpox and survived the local smallpox epidemic. In 1805, to test his claim to have predated Jenner's discovery, Jesty was called before a board of the Original Vaccine Pock Institute in London and was administered smallpox to see whether he would develop the disease.[3]

Several years before, in 1768, a local Berkeley Vale surgeon named John Fewster had also made a scientific connection between both diseases. Writing many years later, he claims that his attempts to variolate some local patients against smallpox had failed.

> At length the cause of the failure was discovered from the case of a farmer who was inoculated several times ineffectually, yet he assured us that he had never suffered the Small Pox, but, says he, "I have had the Cow Pox lately to a violent degree, if that's any odds." We took the hint, and, on enquiry, found that those who were uninfectable had undergone the Cow Pox.[4]

It has recently been argued that Jenner most likely heard about the connection between the two diseases around this time and went on to obsess over the idea for the next thirty years.[5]

From 1770 to 1773, Jenner worked and studied under Dr. George Hardwicke in London, a man who devoted most of his time to experimentation. His methods would certainly have had a profound influence on the life and direction of the young Dr. Jenner. After turning down an offer to accompany Captain Cook's second voyage of exploration, Jenner returned to Berkeley to practice medicine.

A generation would pass by before Jenner would finally test his interest in cowpox inoculation. In 1796, a smallpox epidemic swept across England, killing an estimated thirty-five thousand people.[6] The young doctor was perhaps motivated as much by concern for his patients as by the interests of scientific experimentation. Jenner himself had received variolation at the age of eight, a somewhat effective, though invasive, process. One biographer recounts the following:

> This preparation lasted six weeks. He was bled to ascertain whether his blood was fine; was purged repeatedly, till he became emaciated and feeble; was kept on a very low diet. . . . After this barbarism of human veterinary practice, he was removed to one of the usual inoculation stables, and haltered up with others in a terrible state of disease.[7]

His own experience with the successful but dangerous practice of variolation undoubtedly helped to push him to embrace vaccination. The traditional story unfolds that in May of 1796, a local milkmaid named Sarah Nelms came to visit the doctor. She had recently been infected with cowpox and was complaining about the itching associated with the minor condition. Seeking to test his theory, Jenner subsequently used material from her pockmark to infect a local eight-year-old boy, James Phipps. Phipps seems to have developed a minor reaction to the process, successfully contracting cowpox. He was reported as fully healthy only ten days later. A month and a half later, the doctor tested James to see if he could be infected with smallpox. Phipps did not contract the disease.

Jenner's breakthrough, while mimicking the work of Jesty and Fewster, was to become instrumental because of what he did afterward. His initial attempts to contact the Royal Society proved fruitless. A lack of evidence and a failure to accurately document his experiment caused his claims to be rejected. So instead, Jenner published his *An Inquiry into the Causes and Effects of Variolae Vaccinae: A Disease Discovered in Some of the Western*

Counties of England in 1798. The pamphlet soon spread across the British world. He subsequently journeyed to London to perform vaccinations on others as a method by which to demonstrate his success but was unable to find willing subjects.[8]

Indeed, the initial reaction to Jenner alternated between skepticism and hostility. Religious antagonism continued in the same vein that it had with variolation but was now buttressed by the use of animal material for the injections. Cartoons of the time depicted people with the heads of cows after getting vaccinated, which certainly served to raise public uneasiness. Scientifically, some doubted the veracity of Jenner's methods or questioned the connection between the two diseases. Finally, the lucrative variolation industry saw vaccination as a threat to its monopoly and reacted harshly. All of these elements that were hostile to the process would again be observed in Latin America following Balmis's arrival there.

Despite these multiple avenues of fierce opposition and Jenner's preference for continuing his private practice, vaccination ultimately triumphed, largely because of his pamphlet. The document was widely read, and soon other practitioners began to employ cowpox as a preventative inoculation against smallpox. Hundreds of independent scientists were essentially peer reviewing his work and disseminating it throughout the nation. By 1799, the practice, or at least knowledge of it, had crossed over to Europe. A French doctor by the name of Colon quickly published an essay on the subject in 1800, and most subsequent Spanish treatises are based on his and other French works.[9]

Jenner, despite being finally lauded as a great scientist and hero of the age, preferred to focus on his patients in Berkeley. He soon returned to his practice and even had a small hut built on the ground, which he called the Temple of Vaccinia, where he provided free immunizations to the poor. Apart from popularizing the method by which to rid the world of smallpox, he also helped to start a public health revolution. Variolation was officially outlawed in 1840, and Jenner's method of inoculation subsequently took the world by storm.

Jenner can be better viewed as a prophet who preceded those who acted, a John the Baptist to a later Jesus. The man who built on Jenner's prophesizing and carried the message of vaccination across the globe was Francisco Javier de Balmis. Born on December 2, 1753, only four years after Jenner, Balmis grew up in the city of Alicante. Holding around fourteen thousand people, the town was a center of coastal trade in the region of Valenica. His father was Antonio Balmis y Bas, a skilled surgeon and master of phlebotomy, and his mother was Luisa Berenguer y Nicolini.[10] The family lived on Calle Balseta, a small street situated on the slopes of Alicante, overlooking the sea. Francisco was the second of ten children, which included his older brother Tomas Luis (1751), Juan Bautista (1755), Micaela Gertrudis (1758), Teresa Antonia (1760), Josefa Antonia (1762), Maria Dolores (1764), Tomas Antonio Jose (1765), Maria Manuela (1767), and Jose Francisco (1769). His family had worked as barbers and bloodletters for at least two generations, the medieval equivalent of minor surgeons, a profession that Francisco would initially engage in as well.

At the age of seventeen, in the year 1770, Balmis entered the military hospital of Alicante, where he hoped to train as an army surgeon. Over the course of the next five years, he learned how to perform surgery directly from Dr. Ramón Gilabert.[11] As was common in the profession, the young doctor joined the military expedition sailing for Algeria in 1775. Organized by Count Alexander O'Reilly and meant to demonstrate the military reforms that accompanied Charles III's political and economic reforms, the expedition sailed in June intent on securing the North African coast. The massive force of some thirty thousand men and almost three hundred ships reached Algiers in July of 1775. Despite the king and O'Reilly's high hopes, the assault was an utter failure, resulting in the loss of almost five thousand men. Days later, the damaged fleet, with hundreds of wounded aboard, limped back into port at Balmis's hometown.

In 1778, while still at Alicante, Balmis was required to prove his blood purity, that he was descended from "clean, old Christian blood, not of the bad races of Moors, Jews, Lutherans, Calvinists, nor of those newly converted to our holy faith. Catholic faith, nor found guilty by the holy tribunal of the Inquisition, nor exercised vile offices."[12] This was an old practice, necessitated by the Reconquista, and a component of gaining public office and climbing the social hierarchy. By the early nineteenth century, it was already becoming more of a formality than an actual genealogical test. Balmis passed the Revalida exam on July 11, in Valencia. The official record states that he was of pure blood and "brown hair with a hole in his beard."[13]

In August of 1778, Balmis completed his training at the age of twenty-four and was officially granted the title of surgeon by the Real Protomedicato, in Valencia. This body had been created by Philip II in the sixteenth century in an effort both to modernize the medical field in Spain and to increase royal power over it.[14] As part of the Bourbon reforms and attempts at scientific absolutism, the protomedicato was exported to Italy and the New World. While certainly contributing greatly to the level of public health in the colonies, its hierarchical structure created another source of friction between Spain and the Americas.

Balmis continued his employment in the military for several years, being assigned to his first regiment in 1779. This was the Zamora Regiment, one of the oldest in the Spanish army, and shortly after, he accompanied it to the Great Siege of Gibraltar. Lasting from June 1779 to February 1783 and coinciding with Spain's efforts in the American Revolution, it was to be the longest siege ever against a point that the Spanish had contended for centuries. Despite heavily outnumbering the British, the Spanish army under Martín de Sotomayor was unable to take the fortress. Thousands of soldiers and sailors were killed in action, and many more succumbed to disease. Balmis undoubtedly would have witnessed as much loss from illness as from the bullets and bayonets of the English. His promotion in April of 1781 to full surgeon certainly shows his dedication and skill.

After two years of active campaigning, Balmis and the Zamora Regiment were sent to the Caribbean to join the war effort there, particularly the marquis of Socorro's campaigns aimed at Great Britain's northern Caribbean possessions. The Spanish in 1781 and 1782 were engaged in assaulting

Pensacola and the Bahamas, eventually capturing both locations despite limited numbers and a dearth of supplies. Part of Balmis's time was spent providing medical assistance to the French sailors and marines of Comte de Grasse's fleet. French losses to the British at Les Saintes and Martinique were particularly heavy, and illness was always a frequent enemy at sea. The young doctor was subsequently sent to New Granada, where yellow fever was decimating the Spanish army in South America. Balmis spent a year treating soldiers around Barranquilla and the Guajira Peninsula, attempting to quell the outbreak and gaining valuable firsthand knowledge of the region, its people, and its epidemiological nature.

After the signing of the Treaty of Paris and the ending of war between Spain and Great Britain, much of the Spanish army was disbanded. Balmis was subsequently moved to Mexico in order to continue his training and to provide medical care to the center of the Spanish overseas empire. Landing first at Havana before proceeding to the mainland, he spent 1783 working as an army surgeon in the region of Veracruz, at the Xalapa hospital. The city and region had remained largely stagnated since the sixteenth century but had recently grown in importance because of the increase in trade in the area that accompanied the Bourbon reforms. By the 1780s, Xalapa even boasted a large cathedral, in addition to the hospital. By March of 1786, Balmis was in Mexico City, serving as a surgeon at the Hospital Amor de Dios. Founded by Fray Juan de Zumárraga in 1540, it was the second-oldest care center in the metropolis. In 1786, Balmis also received a degree from the University of Mexico, completing his studies in science. With an additional endowment of 150 reales a month, Balmis was able to live and work comfortably in the region and exploit his natural passion for scientific discovery.

His scientific studies meshed well with his medical pursuits and soon led him to the same types of naturalistic exploration that had been popular with many doctors in both Spain and New Spain during that century. During the early 1790s, while serving as director of the Sala de Galicia Hospital in San Andrés Tuxtla, Mexico, Balmis became interested in testing whether local plants could treat or cure syphilis. He had risen to the position of chief surgeon of the venereal wards after the resignation of Joachín Pío de Eguía y Muro because of financial malfeasance. Balmis actively sought to move beyond traditional methods of treating these types of illnesses.[15] He claims that a local healer named Nicolas Varna, often referred to as El Beato, had heard from a Native woman that certain local plants were being used to effectively treat syphilis. The disease had risen to prominence in Europe in the sixteenth century and had done much to devastate the population of Spain politically and socially.

Balmis chose to focus on agave and begonia, both native to New Spain. The Spanish surgeon examined the various recipes and experimented with them, removing only "the viper meat, as it is no more nutritious than that of chicken."[16] His efforts to champion the Beato Method even found favor with local church officials and the Royal Medical Board of Mexico City. Chief among the supporters was the archbishop of the city himself, Alonso Núñez de Haro y Peralta, who commissioned the physician to bring evidence of his cure to royal officials in Madrid.[17] When Balmis returned to Spain in January of 1792, he brought with him 2,500 pounds of agave and over 700 pounds of begonia. Though his subsequent experiments undertaken in July of 1792 in the various royal hospitals of Madrid proved to be less than encouraging, he did receive the honor of having his name applied to the species that was returned, *Begonia balmisiana.*[18] Balmis also studied and wrote extensively on the nature and treatment of leprosy, dispatching a paper on the topic to the Royal Medical Academy in Madrid. Additionally, upon his return to the Iberian Peninsula, Balmis was appointed as a surgical consultant to the army and was made a royal surgeon as well, receiving an annual salary of 18,000 reales.[19] In 1798, he received yet another medical degree, this one from the University of Toledo. He thereafter continued his scientific research, completing a work entitled *Treatise on the Benefits of Agave and Begonia* in 1794.

Interestingly, his achievements during this episode were to be tarnished by a dispute with Dr. Daniel O'Sullivan. An Irish surgeon, O'Sullivan was educated in France before finishing his studies in Spain. By the late 1780s, O'Sullivan was living and delivering medical care in Mexico. It seems that a confrontation arose between the two men regarding the effectiveness of the Beato Method. While Balmis grew to support the cure following his various tests, O'Sullivan remained a harsh opponent. Worse yet, the Irish physician wrote several tracts personally attacking the Spanish doctor, lambasting his methods and his personal relations. He considered Balmis a charlatan in terms of medical knowledge and questionable in terms of morality because of his "penchant for actresses, in particular one Antonia San Martin, who it would seem was treated by O'Sullivan for venereal disease."[20] The veracity of O'Sullivan's claims matter less than does the pattern it establishes, one that we will see again during Balmis's time in San Juan. The physician often experienced conflict with other doctors and local officials. Some of this was due to jealousy of his accomplishments, while some of it resulted from his own penchant for aggressively pushing his opinion and methods.

In 1797, Balmis was called back to New Spain at the request of the viceroy, Miguel de la Grúa Talamanca, to serve as chief surgeon. His renown in both Mexico and Spain would have made Balmis a reasonable choice for this position. Balmis did not remain long in the New World because of Talamanca's corruption and removal from office shortly after the doctor's arrival. By 1799, Balmis was already back in Spain, having accompanied the viceroy's wife on the return voyage. In the short time he was in the region, Balmis traveled to Caracas and Cumaná in New Granada. An epidemic of yellow fever had erupted in the area of northern South America, killing thousands, and the royal surgeon proceeded there to help treat the sick. The famed naturalist and explorer Alexander von Humboldt had been granted permission by the Spanish crown to perform his own expedition to the region, arriving at the end of the epidemic.[21]

Balmis's involvement with Jenner's discovery began early in 1801. As previously mentioned, the discovery reached the Continent in 1799, most likely arriving in France first, though an abstract appeared in the Spanish journal *Semanario de Agricultura y Artes* in March of 1799.[22] Various Spanish physicians began translating works by Jenner and Colon, while others pushed the practice in letters and essays. In the former group was Dr. Francisco Piquellem, while Pedro Hernandez, Francisco Cano, and D. Vicente Martinez published, respectively, "Origin, Discovery, and Progress of the Inoculation of Vaccine," "An Answer to Objections that Are Made to the New Inoculation of Vaccine," and "Historical and Practical Treatise upon Vaccination." On June 26, 1801, the *Gazeta de Madrid* carried an article about Jenner and vaccination, which Balmis undoubtedly read shortly after its publication. The French physician Jacques-Louis Moreau de La Sarthe also wrote his *Traité Historique et Pratique de la Vaccine* in 1801. The book was dedicated to Jenner as the "benefactor of humanity" and detailed his discovery.[23] Balmis worked to translate the book only months after it was published, and his version was soon available throughout the Spanish world by 1803.[24] Interestingly, the work was dedicated to the mothers of all families, not only because of their sorrow at losing children to smallpox but perhaps hoping to emotionally invest them in the process of vaccination. The royal surgeon himself engaged heavily in administering vaccinations while overseeing several hospitals in Madrid, helping to put Jenner's idea into practice.

Jenner's work and his subsequent publication attracted worldwide interest in smallpox vaccination as a viable medical practice. Likewise, Balmis's own interest in the process and his translation of Moreau's treatise brought the practice to the attention of the Spanish court. When combined with the Enlightenment and absolutist tendencies present in the Bourbon government, the stage was set for the great vaccination expedition. All that was needed was an immediate catalyst.

CHAPTER 6

Surgeons, Smallpox, Sovereigns, and Organizing the Expedition

We've come up against the church, Sancho.

—DON QUIXOTE

THOUGH SMALLPOX WAS AN ACKNOWLEDGED global killer and threat to the Spanish Empire, and Jenner and others had proven that vaccination was possible and cost effective, it would still take a number of divergent events to catalyze the launching of the expedition. Don Quixote's famous statement above accurately describes the many barriers that stood in the way of such an undertaking. Popular fear, local government resistance, geographic and climatic constraints, economic concerns, the ongoing French Revolution, religious questions, and the Byzantine intricacies of the Spanish court all could have delayed or destroyed the attempt at vaccinating the empire. In this instance it would take the efforts of Francisco Balmis, the outbreak of yet another epidemic in the New World, the interest of Viceroy Mendinueta, the Napoleonic invasions, and the personal health history of the Habsburgs to effect the greatest philanthropic expedition in human history. Only Spain at the turn of the nineteenth century possessed these needed catalysts to propel the launching of such a monumental undertaking.

NEW SPAIN

As has been shown, disease was hardly a new event in the Spanish colonies. The land from Mexico to Argentina was periodically ravaged by epidemics, while several other illnesses were endemic to it. From the first smallpox outbreak following the arrival of the Spanish to the Matlazanhuatl Epidemic of 1737, disease limited population growth, challenged local economies, tested the rule of various administrations, and provoked rebellions.

Outbreaks of smallpox were especially feared because of its high mortality rate as well as its historical connections to the decline of the Indigenous population. One of the more dangerous eruptions of smallpox occurred around Mexico City in 1779. First appearing in August of that year, the illness soon expanded out of control, and by October, local authorities realized that a major epidemic had broken out. Though a number of hospitals existed in the city, most notably the Hospital de San Juan de Dios and the Hospital Nuestra Señora de Belén, they soon became overwhelmed by the sheer number of sick and dying. The directors of the buildings appealed to the local government and were granted 23,000 pesos for additional beds, supplies, and food. Likewise, the College of San Andrés, which had been taken from the Jesuits and repurposed as a military barracks, was given back to the Church for use as a hospital for the poor during the outbreak. Archbishop Alonso Núñez de Haro y Peralta quickly set up the building to serve the sick, eventually outfitting it with three hundred beds. This specialized hospital aimed solely at treating smallpox victims, while not unprecedented, still showed the level of concern and organization prevalent at the time in New Spain.[1] Clearly, local civic authorities had learned much from the outbreak of 1737 and quickly moved to provide aid and leadership as smallpox spread across the viceroyalty.

Local physicians employed the most current techniques, though the severity of the outbreak soon led to several rather unorthodox proposals. José Ignacio Bartolache, a Criollo physician who had edited the *Mercurio Volante* from 1772 to 1773, published a pamphlet entitled *An Instruction Which Can Serve to Cure the Sufferers of Epidemic Smallpox.* The tractate leaned heavily on miasmic thinking and recommended the use of bonfires, cannons, and church bells to drive away putrid air while soothing music is played for the infected. Conversely, Dr. Esteban Morel proposed providing variolation to stop the epidemic from spreading, a move that Bartolache eventually supported as well.

Bartolache's life and career represented the dreams and ambitions of many in the Spanish imperial system. Though from a poor family, he had risen up through education to become a respected physician and member of society. He attended both the Jesuit-run College of San Ildefonso and the National Autonomous University of Mexico and graduated with a degree in medicine. Trained in Enlightenment thinking and Italian medical notions, he undoubtedly saw himself as equal to Spanish physicians such as Balmis, who often looked down on colonial medical practitioners.[2]

The local Spanish government, under the control of Viceroy Martín de Mayorga, orchestrated a thorough and pragmatic approach to dealing with the outbreak. Mayorga had only recently been appointed to the position, arriving in August after having served as captain general of Guatemala from 1773 to 1779. In his prior office, Mayorga had organized the region's response to the devastating earthquake of 1773 and was thus experienced with responding to natural disasters. Recommendations for both extreme and more traditional methods were brought into action. The city was subdivided into wards to track and treat the sick more easily. Government officials soon compiled lists of the poor who would need financial support in the event they became ill. Having experienced the pecuniary cost of civic destruction during the Guatemala earthquake of 1773, Mayorga asked for public donations to fund the fight against smallpox, raising an astonishing 147,263 pesos in the process.[3] Cemeteries were set up for mass burials, streets were cleaned, and bonfires were lit around the capital in keeping with Bartolache's recommendations. At the same time, Morel was allowed to operate a variolation clinic within a city hospital.

Mayorga's decision regarding variolation was revolutionary in its impact on public health in the region. The practice was heavily debated by the civil and medical authorities in New Spain, not on religious grounds but largely on scientific ones. It stood in sharp contrast with the experiences of

Cotton Mather, who, in Massachusetts Bay Colony in 1721, found himself in the middle of a religious debate on the issue that quickly turned violent. Some physicians and officials in Mexico City feared that the method was dangerous, would produce unnecessary deaths, and could lead to a larger outbreak. Mayorga, after hearing all sides, finally approved of the practice, allowing Morel to set up a clinic at the Hospital de San Juan de Dios in October. Unfortunately, after all these struggles, few residents actually appeared at his facility to be inoculated. As Morel himself later explained, "The innate repugnance of those who were naturally healthy to voluntarily contract a sickness by artificial means . . . served to persuade the people that they need not be inoculated."[4] Likewise, official efforts to convince the sick to isolate themselves outside of the city largely failed, as the vast majority of the poor saw the lazarettos, or quarantine stations, as merely death houses far away from family and friends.[5]

In the end, it is estimated that around eighteen thousand citizens died during this smallpox epidemic, out of perhaps ninety thousand stricken with the disease.[6] Apart from the devastating loss of life, however, the epidemic of 1779 introduced important public health developments within the region. In addition to Mayorga's revolutionary approval of variolation and the institution of common-sense epidemiological practices, another hospital was opened in the city and distant burial grounds were established for future eruptions of disease. Thus, the outbreak saw a furthering of the actions of the civil government in 1737, an evolution that would continue until Balmis's arrival.

Much credit must go to the various royally appointed officials whose thought appears to have been thoroughly grounded in Enlightenment thinking. The archbishop of Mexico City, Alonso Núñez de Haro y Peralta, had been educated at the University of Toledo and the University of Bologna, eventually earning a doctorate from the latter institution. After serving for several years as a professor and rector at Bologna, he was named archbishop of Mexico in 1772. For the next twenty-eight years he focused on improving both the religious and public health dimensions of New Spain.

Perhaps his greatest contribution was the founding of the Hospital de San Andrés and the reorganization of the Hospital Amor de Dios. Specifically, he worked toward treating and preventing smallpox and syphilis. Finally, it was Núñez de Haro who authorized Sessé's botanical garden during his visit to the region in 1788. The archbishop was not alone in his views, as the concurrent senior judges of the audiencia were like-minded thinkers. All of these men were appointees of Charles III and were well grounded in Enlightenment thinking.[7]

Finally, as previously mentioned, the various viceroys of the era, whether appointed by Charles III or Charles IV, tended to have similar proactive views regarding public health. Chief among these men were Martín de Mayorga Ferrer (1779–83), who battled the smallpox epidemic of 1779 and worked to clean the streets and waterways in Mexico City; Bernardo de Gálvez (1785–86), who worked to relieve a massive typhus outbreak and sponsored further botanical expeditions; Archbishop Núñez (1787), whose accomplishments are discussed in the preceding paragraphs; Miguel de la Grúa Talamanca (1794–98), who instituted numerous reforms during the epidemic of 1797–98; and Juan Vicente de Güemes (1789–94), who did much to improve public sanitation in the capital and encouraged the Malaspina Expedition. These were men who were born and educated in Enlightenment Spain, had military or religious backgrounds, and concerned themselves with the improvement of the cities and people of New Spain.

Even in the borderlands of the Spanish Empire, local public health efforts tended to be extremely modern for the time period. An outbreak of smallpox in the region of Bexar, modern-day San Antonio, in 1786 was responded to with an intense variolation campaign. Domingo Cabello y Robles, the governor of Texas, wrote to Teodoro de Croix, the commander general of the Internal Provinces of the north, as early as 1780 concerning the plight of the Indigenous peoples.

> Indians are being decimated to a degree inexpressible. And so an endless number of them, now apostates, now heathens, have come to these missions, which have been inundated with such people.

But their coming to the missions is not saving these people from nevertheless dying in great numbers. Since they have the custom of abandoning victims in the place where they die, leaving the victims horses and whatever else they owned, I feel that some new plague may arise from so many bodies of Indians.[8]

Cabello went on to suggest that he would immediately take vigorous action to enforce the proper disposal of bodies.

Six years later, Jacobo de Ugarte y Loyola, who had replaced Croix, approved Cabello to undertake a variolation campaign as well.[9] Modeled after those being used in the rest of New Spain, the campaign was designed to reduce the potential for epidemics and relied heavily on close cooperation among local practitioners, state government, and the Church. The governor subsequently communicated with Captain Luis Cazorla and his minister of justice to carry out the task.[10] Public health in the Spanish Empire was not confined to a particular racial group or class, as the ability of disease to cross socioeconomic boundaries was now well understood.

Despite these reformers and their reforms, disease continued to plague the region. In 1786, a massive famine erupted in New Spain that was followed by an outbreak of typhus. The combined events killed an estimated three hundred thousand people in the region. Then smallpox returned to devastate the capital in 1797, killing seven thousand residents and sickening sixty-three thousand more. In April of 1796, the ship *La Bentura* docked in Acajutla, on the Pacific coast, in modern-day El Salvador, after sailing from Callao in Peru. Smallpox-infected passengers and crew were discovered onboard, and the vessel was placed under quarantine. Despite this, outbreaks of the disease continued and were reported in Oaxaca and Acapulco by July. Though it is difficult to trace the origins of the illness directly back to the *La Bentura*, the ship remains a possible vector. Following this latest outbreak, which occurred during Talamanca's administration, public health efforts reached new heights in the region.

Viceroy Talamanca took decisive action by July 1796, issuing a series of rules and memorandums, many of them based on policies that had been used previously during other outbreaks. Chief among these were isolating the sick, burying the dead far from the city, banning trade with infected areas, and calling for voluntary variolation. Despite these measures, however, the disease continued to progress, and by the end of 1796, it was reported throughout Oaxaca and Zacatecas. With the capital city surrounded, it was only a matter of time before that barrier was breached and the residents of Mexico City fell victim to the pestilence.

On February 28, 1797, in consolation with the audiencia, the viceroy issued a further list of regulations.

1. The sick were to be isolated in remote lazarettos in an opposite direction from prevailing winds.
2. New cases were to be reported to civil and church authorities.
3. Mexico City was to be subdivided into smaller zones and patrolled for the infected.
4. A cordon sanitaire was to be created around the capital.
5. Approaches to the city were to be guarded and all those entering or leaving inspected.
6. Bonfires were to be lit to drive away the illness.
7. All incoming mail was to be smoked.
8. Voluntary variolation was to be encouraged.
9. Public charity to fund the poor who were ill was to be encouraged.
10. Burials were to take place at a distance from the city.
11. Public and private prayer was to be encouraged.
12. In extreme cases, public buildings and funds could be appropriated by judges.
13. All other ideas should be reported to the viceroy.

While not revolutionary in nature, the ideas were a thorough collection of current and time-tested methods for dealing with large-scale pestilence.

The most vulnerable groups bristled at several of the suggestions. The poor tended to resent the notion of being removed to isolation centers, seeing them as places of death or as a way to expel the poor from the city. Many still opposed inoculation for personal or scientific reasons, and the dispute was once again taken up by the protomedicato. Resistance to the measures put forth by the government served to worsen the outbreak and increase casualties.

This particular outbreak was also worsened by the Wars of the First and Second Coalition, then raging in Europe. Regardless of whether Spain was fighting with or against France, the cost of the various conflicts weighed heavily on the country's national budget. Much-needed funds were diverted from the Spanish colonies, and due in part to this, the various hospitals of Mexico City became overwhelmed and underfunded. In response, Talamanca organized the Junta Principal de Caridad in October 1797. Both public and private charity was sought to finance the fight against smallpox. Within a month, $58,000 had been pledged by private groups and government institutions, while the viceroyalty itself contributed $69,000.[11]

By December of 1798, the epidemic began to subside and was officially declared over on January 18, 1798. In the end, some 7,000 people died of smallpox, around 10 percent of those infected. Overall, around 50 percent of the city's population of 135,000 people was stricken with the disease—the vast majority being perhaps from the younger generation, born after the previous outbreak.[12] While the loss of life was profound, its impact on the economics of the region and the already-strained social problems was much more devastating. There was substantially more poverty in the capital in 1797 than in 1779 because of a variety of factors, not the least of which were the smallpox and typhus outbreaks that struck the region. Donald Cooper estimates that from 1761 to 1813, five major epidemics struck Mexico City alone, causing at least 50,000 deaths.[13] When the number of sick is added into these figures and the loss of production and economic growth included, it becomes evident that illness remained the greatest threat to the development of the region. For Mexico City, frequent epidemics and low immigration meant that its population would take until almost 1800 to recover to the level it had been in 1500. Disease was weakening the Spanish Empire and catalyzing revolution.

Despite this, the Spanish imperial government could be somewhat satisfied with its handling of these epidemics. The "Hispanic tradition of government charity which . . . proved reasonably effective and certainly merciful" had helped to mitigate the 1797 outbreak.[14] The actions undertaken by the viceroy, the Church, and the local government resulted in a low death rate compared to previous outbreaks. The latest ideas of the Enlightenment had been followed, and over three thousand individuals had been voluntarily variolated. This last piece proved to be especially important when Balmis arrived, as there was at least a tacit acceptance of the practice of medical intervention in the region.

By comparison, the contemporaneous yellow fever epidemic that hit Philadelphia in 1793 produced much more panic and loss of life. While Mayor Matthew Clarkson, who was ill at the time, remained behind to organize relief efforts, most of the city council fled, and the state government ended its session early. Almost half the population of the city joined the government in withdrawing from Philadelphia, making the five-thousand-person death toll statistically higher than the 10 percent of the city's population it officially represented. Treatment split along political lines, socioeconomic and racial disparities were worsened, and cooperation between the states in the region proved wanting.

GUATEMALA

The 1779 smallpox outbreak in New Spain moved southward as well, eventually reaching the audiencia of Guatemala by 1780. Local civic leaders employed similar tactics to those used farther north but also leaned heavily on the practice of variolation. Dr. José Flores, who taught medicine at the University of San Carlos and later produced most of the recommendations for the Balmis Expedition, was one of the early proponents of variolation.

Working with Matías de Gálvez, the captain-general of the province, and with the approval of local church officials, Flores was able to inoculate thousands of people starting in June of 1780.

In contrast with the general view held elsewhere, especially in Philadelphia during the yellow fever outbreak, that the poor were vectors for illness and should be helped only in order to protect the wealthy, city officials in Guatemala portrayed the inoculation campaign in terms of moral compassion: "It is very grave for them, and we can only give them compassion and tenderness."[15] Clearly elements of traditional Catholic belief as well as new thinking inherent in the Enlightenment were at work here.

Flores's campaign appears to have been remarkably successful. He records that by August 22, 1780, he had personally overseen the variolation of 200 people, of whom only 1 would go on to die.[16] Considering that around the same time period, 8,667 were sick with smallpox in the capital city alone, many of whom perished, Flores's efforts, though small in scale, certainly helped to combat the epidemic and set an example for future practices.

The key to his success was what he saw as his own unique method of delivering the vaccine to Indigenous villages. Laying out his method in his writings, he advised, "Take extreme care not to use violence and not to terrify the Indians."[17] Flores sought as much as possible to mollify the fears and superstitions of the Indigenous peoples as well as to rely on local products and techniques, arguing that Spanish medical equipment could often be frightening to the uneducated villagers of the countryside. He would later go on to argue that employing church officials and lending an air of the divine to the practice would also help to convince the Indigenous people to receive variolation.[18] His methods and ideas seem to reflect traditional Jesuit practices of dealing with local populations and were almost certainly influenced by them.

By the time of the next major outbreak in the region in 1794, Flores had been elevated to the position of protomedicato of the audiencia. In this office, he was able to push more widespread variolation on the population of the region. Once more, the doctor leaned heavily on local churches to aid the process, either in blessing and promoting the undertaking or in serving as translators to the local population. Thanks to his focus on creating a cordon sanitaire, his effective education of physicians through a detailed manual, and his employment of local clergy, Flores was able to save thousands of lives and open up the region to future vaccination campaigns. His later recounting of his welcome at one of the villages to which he traveled showed the thankfulness of the local population: "I was not received as before, but with the ringing of bells and the throwing of flowers. . . . They raised their hands to heaven and, in their unpolished style, gave thanks to the king for saving the life of their children."[19]

The process of variolation would gather additional support in New Spain around the same time, while experiencing varying levels of support elsewhere in the empire. Interestingly, the practice seems to have entered the region of Chile, where it was allegedly introduced by Friar Pedro Manuel Chaparro in the 1760s, slightly earlier than it reached Mexico. It was introduced to Peru in 1778.[20] In the case of Peru, introduction of the practice followed the publication in 1776 of Cosme Bueno's work on the subject. A local friar in Peru variolated a patient in 1778, only to have the process roundly attacked and discredited shortly afterward. The practice would not gain a permanent foothold in the viceroyalty until the 1790s, after the use of it in New Spain and New Grenada produced such positive results.

The outbreak of 1796 exposed the dangers of disease in the region of New Spain, a lesson that officials feared could be repeated and magnified elsewhere. Not everyone accepted the public health practices being pushed by the elites in Mexico City. When smallpox appeared in the small town of Teotitlán del Valle, fifteen miles from the capital of Oaxaca, civic officials and medical personnel put in place the standard modern solutions to disease management. The sick were isolated, makeshift hospitals were constructed, and roadblocks to neighboring towns were put up. Unfortunately, these actions infuriated the public as they strangled the economy of a market town whose citizens made their living off the export of fabrics.

The situation appears to have been worsened by stark socioeconomic divides between the Criollo leadership of the town and the largely Indigenous population. Anger flared when people attempted to leave the village and mothers sought to seize their children who had been forced into the infirmary. The situation finally produced a full-scale riot as women stoned and then stormed the church, demanding that a recently deceased child be buried there rather than in the special cemetery recently established outside of the town for victims of the pestilence. As one observer recounted, "The Indians had built the church and that they were not animals, to be buried in the countryside."[21] In the end, local residents triumphed, and officials removed much of the machinery of quarantine and public health management. Though an isolated incident, the protest was reflective of the need to better educate the populace and of the extremes to which scientific absolutism led civic authorities to feel they could control the population.

NEW GRANADA

South America witnessed many of the same epidemics and efforts to combat them as did the Caribbean and New Spain. At the same time, South America's historically smaller population led to immigration schemes, many of which involved the poor and sickly of Spain, bringing and spreading illness to the New World. In one particular episode, which took place in 1778, over 1,900 peasants were recruited from Asturias and Castile to move to Patagonia. The poor health of many of the participants forced the Spanish government to set up various public health services to save the scheme from total failure.[22] In keeping with the similar pattern that developed in the territory of New Spain, it was the Enlightenment era–trained viceroys who helped to push advances in public health and sanitation that did much to alleviate the suffering of the people.

José Solís Folch de Cardona, whose administration lasted from 1753 to 1761, ran the gamut from notoriety to piety during his time in office. Despite this, he worked diligently to reform medical care in the region. As part of his efforts, he endowed the chair of medicine at the Colegio el Rosario and set up the Hospital San Juan de Dios. The university was established in 1653 and soon became a leading center of medical studies in South America. Finally, Cardona had to contend with a massive outbreak of smallpox that burned across the region in 1761, killing thousands in Caracas alone.[23]

De Cardona was followed by Pedro Messía de la Cerda, who held office from 1761 to 1773, and Manuel de Guirior, who was in power from 1773 to 1776. De la Cerda worked extensively to aid the Mutis Expedition as it explored the region, embracing its mission and appreciating its contributions. Interestingly, Mutis himself had taught at the Colegio del Rosario during the 1760s and most likely had political connections already in the region. De Guirior helped to establish yet another hospital in the capital, a feat he would repeat on a larger scale while overseeing the Viceroyalty of Peru from 1776 to 1780. Finally, Antonio Caballero y Góngora, who was viceroy from 1782 to 1789, saw his time in office overwhelmed by a series of epidemics. From 1782 to 1783, smallpox ravaged the northern coast, killing thousands. The epidemic led to calls for medical reforms and introduced variolation to the region.[24] It was around this time that the region also saw the worst outbreak of measles in a century. Lasting from 1785 to 1788, the importance of this episode rests in the impact it had on the future of Latin American independence. One of the victims of the disease was a young Simón Bolívar, who was sterilized as a result of his illness.[25] Much like his idol George Washington, who suffered from a similar issue, Bolívar's inability to produce an heir may have driven him more toward republicanism and away from offers to accept a crown after the revolution against Spanish rule.

Of even greater importance was Viceroy Pedro Mendinueta y Múzquiz, who oversaw the region from 1797 to 1803. Mendinueta had a military background, having served in various Spanish wars for almost forty years. Perhaps because of his experience with disease on the battlefield, he became heavily involved in promoting public health initiatives upon arriving in Bogotá. As with other viceroys, he worked cooperatively with the various observatory expeditions that crossed his province, including Alexander von

Humboldt's in 1801. At the same time, he worked extensively with Mutis to improve medical studies at the city's university, which included the first dissections of cadavers to be undertaken in South America. This stands in sharp contrast with medical school practices in New York City, where rumors of Columbia University students robbing graves led to a riot in 1788 that killed twenty people and injured John Jay and Baron von Steuben. Finally, Mendinueta went about reorganizing the Hospital San Juan de Dios, providing for monthly inspections and handing out medicine to the poor.

Overall, the leaders of the various viceroyalties were heavily concerned with local epidemics and efforts to improve public health. Part of this concern emerged from the ideals of the Enlightenment, which concerned itself with proper social order and the well-being of the population. Traditional Catholic notions and the role of the Church in organizing health care and medical relief efforts also continued at this time. Fears of civil unrest spurred by famines and fever drove more aggressive government action. Finally, the ultimate role of the colonies as the economic backbone of the Spanish Empire led local and national leaders to call for the region's development, a development that was severely hindered by endemic disease.

BOURBONS AND SMALLPOX

As with their Habsburg predecessors, the Bourbon family was touched by disease generally and by smallpox specifically. This personal connection would do much to convince Charles IV to move against the illness. As previously mentioned, Charles II's mental and physical sickness helped to bring down the Habsburg dynasty in Spain and led to the War of the Spanish Succession that followed. In an attempt to avoid this outcome, the king and the royal court in Madrid agreed in 1696, and reaffirmed in 1698, that Joseph Ferdinand, son of the elector of Bavaria, would take the throne. In 1699, as Charles II's health deteriorated even further, Ferdinand was brought to Brussels to prepare for the journey to Madrid. Unfortunately, the six-year-old boy was struck suddenly with smallpox and died in February.[26] His death threw the succession into dispute once again and, following Charles's death a year later, produced the War of the Spanish Succession.

Though the Bourbon dynasty was politically stronger than the Habsburg dynasty had been, it too suffered from disease, particularly smallpox. Philip V produced ten children from his two marriages. Of these offspring, those of his first marriage were visited the most by illness. His eldest son and heir, Louis, briefly became king in 1724 upon the abdication of his father. But only eight months after rising to the throne, he was struck down by smallpox. After fainting in church in the middle of August, Louis was brought home to his palace, where his condition worsened. Every possible measure was taken to heal the young monarch, including bringing dozens of holy relics into his bedroom. One such treasure involved items sacred to San Diego of Alcalá.[27] The Franciscan lay brother had performed missionary work in the Canary Islands before helping to treat an outbreak of illness during a pilgrimage to Rome in 1520. His entire body had been brought to the room of Don Carlos, the son of Philip II, following an accident that left him temporarily paralyzed.[28] Despite these attempts at divine intervention, Louis succumbed to smallpox on August 31, 1724, returning his father to the throne. Louis's brother Philip died shortly after birth, while Philip Peter Gabriel fell to disease at the age of seven. Though Philip V's final son by his first marriage, Ferdinand VI, rose to the throne in 1746, he was unable to produce an heir. Following the death of his wife Barbara of Portugal in 1758, he fell into depression and died a year later.

Charles IV, who reigned from 1788 to 1808, was particularly affected by the ravages of disease among both his siblings and children. Of his twelve siblings, five died young from various illnesses. His brother Gabriel in particular was hard pressed by smallpox. After the birth of Gabriel's third child in 1788, his wife, Maria Ana Vitoria of Portugal, and their child Carlos fell victim to the disease. At the same time, Charles's elder brother, Felipe, was excluded from the throne because of mental illness, while another brother, Francis, died at the age of fourteen from illness. In fact,

Charles's rise to power was predicated on the winnowing effect of disease on the Bourbon family.

As for his own children, Charles IV and his wife, Maria Luisa of Parma, produced fourteen, of whom only six survived to adulthood. His four sons would all die before the age of three, victims of various infections. Worse yet, in 1794, Charles IV's wife and daughter Maria Teresa were stricken with smallpox. Though Maria Luisa survived the ordeal, her daughter did not, dying on November 2. Both parents were as devastated by this loss as they were the deaths of their other children. In response, the queen urged her husband to variolate their remaining children, a weighty decision because not all survived the process. Though the treatment was successfully carried out, it left their offspring scarred for life from the weaker form of smallpox that they would all suffer from.

Nevertheless, Charles IV became a proponent of inoculation, and in November of 1798 issued a proclamation calling for the entire Spanish population of the empire to be variolated.[29] The roots of this move clearly lay in his economic needs, his concern for the well-being of his people, the need for a healthy and robust population in light of the ongoing wars of the French Revolution, his Catholic faith, the ideas of the Enlightenment and absolutism, and his own personal history with the disease. Though it is difficult to judge the initial result of his order, he continued to be interested in the subject. In 1799, Charles IV received a copy of Jenner's publication from an Italian physician and subsequently issued an additional decree the next year announcing the availability of vaccination throughout the empire.[30] Clearly, the Bourbon monarchs were not opposed to the latest medical discoveries and in many ways were active proponents of them.

1802 EPIDEMIC

Despite the advances in public health care in Latin America, the region was once again struck by smallpox in 1802, an outbreak that would lead directly to the launching of the Balmis Expedition. This particular epidemic most likely began in Cartagena de Indias, before proceeding aboard trade vessels up the Magdalena River and toward the capital of the province. As with previous outbreaks, the local government acted quickly to attempt to halt its spread. On June 12, 1802, the municipal council of Santa Fe issued regulations regarding movement, trade, and public burial and set up isolation hospitals in remote locations. In light of the recent royal proclamations, the council also began to search for available cowpox vaccines to stave off a larger and deadlier outbreak. Unfortunately, supplies of the vaccine proved to be too expensive or too rare to locate in the immediate region.

Some private individuals sought to obtain supplies of Jenner's treatment, but to no avail. José Ignacio de Pombo, one of the wealthiest merchants in Cartagena, tried in 1803 to obtain a supply of vaccination material from North America. He had always been interested in science and medicine, having hosted both Mutis and Humboldt during their respective expeditions to the region.[31] In this case, his concerns stemmed less from scientific curiosity and more from the health of his own children stricken with the disease as well as from the economic impact the outbreak would have on the region. Unfortunately, his efforts proved to be no more successful than those of the council.[32] Though his search was in vain, Pombo later successfully petitioned the government of the viceroyalty to improve medical education in the region, including the construction of an anatomical theater.[33]

At the same time, in Guatemala, José de Córdova and the famed doctor Professor Narciso Esparragosa imported copies of the vaccine from New Orleans, Mexico City, and Havana, but all samples arrived useless.[34] Esparragosa, who had studied under Dr. José Flores, even attempted to create his own vaccine using instructions provided by the Mexican doctor José Mariano Mociño, but to no avail.[35] Finally, an effort by the royal family physician, Dr. Lorenzo Berges, to personally travel to Latin America with the new viceroy of New Spain, José de Iturrigaray, and administer vaccines proved to be completely ineffective. Worse yet, any help that Berges could have offered to Balmis ended with his subsequent death. Doctors and scientists in the region attempted to locate domestic sources of cowpox, and even tested serum derived from sheep, but efforts all ended in failure.[36]

The situation continued to worsen as thousands were sickened and killed by the disease. The governor of Cartagena wrote to the council on November 5, 1803, warning of the "unfortunate situation of the province due to the great ravages of the natural smallpox in the entire kingdom."[37] The disease spread along familiar paths, eventually reaching into the Caribbean and New Spain. Peru was breached around the same time, with official reports claiming that "smallpox spread in Lima and Bogota as a true epidemic that caused many patients to perish, most of them from the indigenous class."[38] A similar letter was received by Charles IV himself, pleading with the king for financial help.

The Venezuelan poet Andrés Bello, an eyewitness to the events, described the situation several years later in terms of biblical pestilence and death in his "Ode to the Vaccine."

> The palace as well as the hut,
> Is covered in mourning;
> The tender child perishes with the mother;
> As does the old man and the young men.
> All civil functions break down;
> The citizen leaves the infected walls of the city;
> Nothing is seen, nothing is heard, but terror, sadness, woes, and laments.
> What spoils are before her chariot?
> Tisiphone!
> What a great number of victims to drag to despair and discouragement.
> How many die from the hardest of abandonments!
> The ties that bind break down:
> The wife flees to the husband, the son to the father
> and the slave to the owner.

One of the more historically important victims of the 1802 epidemic in New Granada was the Salavarrieta family. Of above-average means, the family had moved to Bogotá in the late 1790s and was living comfortably when the pestilence struck. The father and mother were killed, along with two of the eight children. Of those that survived, some joined the Church, while others drifted through various towns doing odd jobs to survive. One of these was Policarpa Salavarrieta, who would go on to become an active participant in the revolution and was famously executed by the Spanish in 1817.

Charles III's reforms had done much to streamline the functions of the royal government, including the Council of the Indies, over which he had placed a secretary of state to expedite its functions. On December 25, 1802, this individual called together the council to discuss the grave situation in New Granada. Charles IV had written to the group querying whether "they believed in the possibility of distributing the vaccine in America and what would be the most appropriate methods to do so."[39] This revolutionary idea alone should be considered his greatest accomplishment and shows Charles IV embracing the latest ideas of the scientific revolution and the Enlightenment. While it is unknown whether the monarch himself independently developed the plan or whether his closest advisers recommended it, his opinion, nevertheless, carried great weight in the council, which eventually favored the idea. Considering Manuel Godoy's dominant position at this point in controlling Spain's politics, support from him was clearly essential for launching the mission. Godoy subsequently devoted several passages in his memoirs to detailing elements of the voyage and its success.[40]

In keeping with the letters from both New Granada and the king, it was decided to investigate possible ways in which Spain could help to mitigate the outbreak and prevent future ones. One of the members of the council, Francisco Requena, who had spent many years serving various political and military roles in the colonies, settled on the idea of bringing vaccinations to the Americas but was unsure how best to proceed.[41] In response, the council decided to contact Dr. José Flores, one of Charles IV's royal court physicians, because of his public health accomplishments in Guatemala.

Flores, a native of Chiapas, had spent considerable time in the colonies and had taught medicine at the University of Guatemala in the 1780s. During his time there, he wrote extensively on a potential cure for cancer, utilizing a native lizard of the region.[42] More importantly though, as previously discussed, he had worked for years inoculating Maya populations throughout the region. In fact, Guatemala's use of variolation predated that of both Mexico and Peru.[43] Flores's concerns were humanitarian as well as practical, as the Indigenous villages that surrounded the audiencia's capital would have allowed for the transmission of the disease to the city.

After being appointed to the Royal Medical Board in 1792, Flores undertook a medical tour of Italy and Spain, making contacts with the leaders in medical treatment and inoculation. While much of what he discovered merely reinforced his preexisting notions regarding the practice of variolation, he was also introduced to new methods of organization. Upon his return to New Spain, he was appointed as the first protomedicato of the audiencia and set about organizing local health institutions to treat and prevent future epidemics. During this time, perhaps thanks in part to the contacts he had made during his tour of Italy and Spain, Flores undoubtedly heard of Jenner's great discovery.

By 1803, Flores was residing in Madrid and eagerly answered the council's call.

> This . . . is the crowning moment of my glory; because it provides me the most happy opportunity to promote an easy and safe method to eradicate smallpox, and forever liberate the inhabitants of those lands from the most frightening contagions. I ask you then to listen to . . . a medical physician who burns for love for his homeland, all of America, all of humanity.[44]

Flores's glowing opening to his report neatly laid out his general view, influenced by Catholic belief and Enlightenment philosophy, regarding man's duty to his fellow man.

His subsequent report to the body on a possible course of action against smallpox detailed the impact of the pestilence on the region and the prospective steps that could be taken by the crown to mitigate the impact. His official account chronicled the history of smallpox in the Americas, paying particular attention to its economic impact as well as to the disproportionate suffering the disease caused Indigenous populations. Flores highlighted the role of the disease in the conquest of the region and discussed the duty of the Bourbon monarch and the Council of the Indies to care for the local population. Clearly, much of this was in keeping with his own twenty-year history of vaccinating Indigenous populations. Flores's manifesto was compelling in that it touched on every possible argument—political, socioeconomic, religious, scientific, and historical—to convince the council to act.

His actual plan of action called for the transport of cowpox vaccination material across the Atlantic to inoculate the general population using every possible means. To ensure the survival of the pathogen, it was to be brought to the Americas on two vessels by three different methods. Live cows and infected children would to be put on ships, and "a portion of the selected pus would be placed between two plates of glass sealed carefully with wax."[45] The hope was that by employing these methods, there was the possibility of at least some of the material making it across the ocean. In addition, the transport of live cows would allow for the establishment of a reservoir of cowpox for future vaccination efforts. Flores recommended that the vaccine be brought by two separate ships, one to Veracruz and one to Cartagena, in order to reach the major population centers of the empire. From these cities it could then be disseminated throughout the region.

Interestingly, Flores spent considerable time highlighting the role religion and the Church would play in the successful inoculation of the people. Realizing that the Church already had an organizational presence within the community and that its support would also counter pseudo-religious and social apprehension toward the practice, the royal physician proposed imbuing the process with sacramental authority.

When a child is taken to be baptized, after administration of the sacrament the priest will advise and persuade the godparents of their obligation to return the child after four to six months, when it is well-fed and healthy, so that it can be vaccinated. In this act, an acolyte bearing a lighted candle and the priest, dressed in surplice and stole, will bless the child and say a prayer. Once concluded, the parish physician or one designated for this purpose or the priest himself, will perform the operation. When finished, the priest will say a prayer and warn the parents that without fail they must bring him news of the child's recovery, to be recorded in the parish registry. This vaccination registry would be stored with the other parish records; the vaccination lymph, if there would be more fresh to be passed from arm to arm, would be carefully stored between two sheets of glass in a separate box in the sacristy, where the chrismatories are kept.[46]

The merging of the vaccination process with preexisting religious ceremonies would not only ensure compliance and recordkeeping but also lend an air of religious authority to the practice. To further legitimize the process, Flores recommended garnering support from the pope by having him promulgate a bull supporting the operation: "Accompanying it with religion, so that the pueblo can venerate it, appreciate it, crave it."

The notion of combining scientific and religious authority harkens back to centuries of tradition in Spain and previous notions from the Renaissance and the Enlightenment. As has been seen, the Church's role in providing medical care and guidance as well as in granting legitimacy to scientific discoveries was well established in the minds of the population. When Dr. Esteban Morel published his work on the benefits of variolation in 1779, he leaned heavily on both Christian notions and Greek mythological imagery. Describing the practice as a gift of Minerva, he sought to utilize traditionally recognized elements to help push the practice on both the learned and the general population.

Requena's and Flores's ideas were certainly influenced by the actions of Dr. Jean de Carro. Shortly after reading about Jenner's discovery, Dr. Carro obtained samples of the vaccine from London and used them in late August of 1799 to successfully inoculate a patient in Vienna. Following his success in the Austrian Empire, he proceeded to help spread the practice through Central and Eastern Europe, even sending samples to the British ambassador in Istanbul.[47] Interestingly, Jenner's work followed the reverse of the path of variolation through the Eastern Hemisphere, clearly showing the shift in power and scientific knowledge that had taken place in the world during the seventeenth and eighteenth centuries. Working with Dr. Luigi Sacco of Italy, Carro then dispatched samples to Baghdad and Bombay. By 1802, vaccinations were even being carried out in various parts of British India.

On March 22, 1803, the Council of the Indies read Flores's report and approved of his overall idea. King Charles IV soon after granted his enthusiastic support as well. Though his ascension in 1788 had been seen as an end to the launching of scientific and exploratory expeditions to the New World, largely because of his own lack of interest and the rising threats posed by the French Revolution, the aforementioned personal and national catalysts drove him to action. According to later reports, the monarch was "filled with compassion and love for his faithful vassals."[48] Discounting for obvious royal propaganda in the statement, the monarch must have borne an active interest in the welfare of his imperial subjects to justify the costs of such an undertaking. Plans were quickly drawn up for an expedition to provide vaccinations to the Spanish subjects of the New World.

The larger problem became how best to transport the vaccine across the Atlantic Ocean in the most effective and inexpensive way. Though Flores's overall plan for the mission had been adopted, his idea of employing cows as a means by which to transmit the vaccine was thought not to be economically viable or even physically feasible.[49] Instead, the council looked for additional ideas and strategies. Francisco Balmis subsequently answered the call of the Royal Medical Board with a radical proposal that built on Flores's notion of using live human subjects. He recommended that the expedition employ two dozen orphans for the purpose of transporting cowpox to the Americas. The illness, and thus the vaccine, would be passed from orphan to orphan as the ships traveled across the ocean. This human daisy chain of pestilence was the surest way to allow for the movement of a live virus. Though the concept was already in use on a smaller scale in various communities then practicing vaccination, the idea of bridging an ocean with it was unheard of. The council enthusiastically approved his proposal and set about laying plans for its execution.

What initially began as a two-pronged offensive aimed at both New Spain and New Granada, with Flores heading one and Balmis the other, was soon altered by the Board of Chamber Surgeons. By May of 1803, it was decided to employ only one vessel, with the entire project headed by Francisco Balmis himself. Once in the New World, Balmis would coordinate with Dr. Berges and then proceed at his own discretion to vaccinate people in both provinces. A royal proclamation was issued on June 28 confirming the appointment and the mission, and it was quickly organized over the next two months. A combination of economic restraint on the part of the council and Balmis's own desire to have full control over the undertaking probably prompted the downsizing of the expedition.

The Balmis Expedition was hardly the effort of one individual man. Instead, the actions of numerous persons, government officials, and medical thinkers from Mexico to Austria helped to formulate and organize what would become perhaps the greatest humanitarian mission in the history of the world. Nor was it the result of one particular episode but instead represented the nexus of several centuries of events, experiences, and thought. The Balmis Expedition truly represented a convergence of human experiences.

CHAPTER 7

Balmis in the Americas

I don't imagine the annals of history furnish an example
of philanthropy so noble, so extensive as this.

—EDWARD JENNER

THE EXPEDITION BEING ORGANIZED BY BALMIS in the summer
of 1803 was destined to battle more than just smallpox. The landscape and
infrastructure of New Spain and New Granada offer insurmountable obsta-
cles to any military or scientific excursion. While the previous undertakings
launched by Charles III could at least proceed at a leisurely pace through
the region, mitigating some of the pressures of geography, weather, and
logistics, time was clearly a factor for Balmis's mission. At the same time,
local civil and religious officials often proved to be unreceptive to the idea
of mass inoculation for a variety of reasons. In addition, local practitioners
often resented the scientific absolutism that Balmis represented, as well
as the potential economic loss resulting from the mission's philanthropic
distribution of the vaccine. Moreover, the local people themselves were
occasionally resistant to the procedure for reasons related to superstition,
government opposition, or lack of knowledge. Clearly, the greatest obstacle
to be faced was whether the live virus would survive the often-unpredict-
able voyage across the Atlantic Ocean.

News soon spread to the general population about the great undertaking. The *Gazeta de Madrid* reported in August that

the beautiful discovery of the vaccine, accredited in Spain and
almost all of Europe as an effective prevention against the virus, has

resulted in the request by the King to spread it to his dominions in the Indies, where usually there is a large number of victims, who are sacrificed to this horrible plague. Therefore, it has been mandated, after hearing the opinion of the Council and many wise men, to form a maritime expedition of qualified practitioners directed by the honorary Physician of the Chamber, Dr. Francisco Xavier de Balmis and paid for by the Royal Treasury.[1]

Copies of the circular were dispatched to the Americas as well, informing the general colonies of the imminent arrival of Balmis and the vaccine. While this was meant to inform and encourage local leaders and the general population, it also produced divisions among them in how best to treat the arrival of the Spanish. At the same time, the news encouraged those seeking to profit from inoculation to hurriedly (and occasionally unsafely) acquire and sell cowpox material themselves.

Balmis began organizing for the expedition on August 24, 1803, in Madrid, two months after official approval to head the undertaking. In total, the crown granted 90,000 reales for fitting out the voyage, with an additional 16,000 reales granted yearly for the upkeep of the mission. As this was also a scientific expedition, it needed to be fitted out with specialized equipment beyond what would normally accompany a transoceanic voyage. Some of the equipment needed included medical chests, two thousand glass plates for vaccines, a pneumatic machine to seal the plates, barometers, thermometers, and blank journals to record vaccinations. The scientific and meteorological equipment was largely brought along to ascertain the impact of temperature and the elements on the vaccine material. Not only was the voyage attempting to bring an experimental method to the colonies, but the entire voyage was effectively an experiment in and of itself.

Perhaps most importantly, the project purchased five hundred copies of Moreau de La Sarthe's book on Jenner's procedures. Balmis hoped to establish local vaccine centers that would do most of the immediate inoculating and promote the practice in the future. His translation of Moreau's treatise would thus serve as their immediate handbook upon his departure. In keeping with the ideas of Flores and others, it was thought that local ignorance was the greatest impediment to improving public health in the region. Therefore, proper education by knowledgeable outsiders was key.

In order to cross the Atlantic, the expedition fitted out the *María Pita*. The choice of ship was not without controversy. Despite the humanitarian nature of the voyage, the owners of the only suitable ships at La Coruña, the four-hundred-ton *Silph* and the two-hundred-ton corvette *María Pita*, demanded extraordinary payments from the royal government.[2] Balmis himself found a cheaper option with the *San José*, which was offered at a price of 2,000 pesos less per month than the other ships.[3] Owned by Manuel de Goicoechea, the ship was due to arrive in early October, allowing for just enough time to repair and refit it before the scheduled departure date in November. Unfortunately, the *San José* failed to appear, and Balmis was forced to purchase the much more expensive *María Pita*. Named for the heroine of the 1589 English attack on La Coruña, the ship was destined to help save many more lives across the ocean.

Apart from material, the mission required an experienced team of doctors, explorers, administrators, and medical professionals. Both the council and Balmis had a hand in nominating members, though the latter worked hard to make sure it was largely composed of persons who would be loyal to him. The initial team was made up of Dr. Francisco Javier de Balmis as the chief physician, José Salvany y Lleopart as his deputy, Ramón Fernández de Ochoa, Manuel Julian Grajales, and Antonio Gutiérrez Robredo as medical aides, and Francisco Pastor y Balmis, Rafael Lozano y Perez, Basilio Bolaños, Àngel Crespo, Pedro Ortega, and Antonio Pastor as nurses and assistants. The majority were accomplished surgeons and scientists and brought decades of medical experience to the undertaking.

José Salvany was a surgeon at the royal residence, having studied medicine and surgery in Barcelona before following a path similar to Balmis's and becoming a military surgeon. While engaged in these duties, Salvany contracted malaria, a disease that would plague him and limit his accomplishments for the remainder of his short life. Manual Julian Grajales was born in 1775 in the province of Toledo and studied at the Royal College of San Carlos as well as at the University of Toledo and was a young but gifted doctor. Antonio Gutiérrez Robredo was born in 1773 and was likewise educated at San Carlos but then followed a military path, serving as a surgeon in the War of the Oranges in Portugal in 1801. Both Lozano and Antonio Pastor, Balmis's nephew, had experience with performing vaccinations and would prove to be trustworthy and useful assistants on the voyage.

The only weakness in the team's cohesion appears to have been the appointment of Ramón Fernández de Ochoa. Not much is known about his background, save for a brief reference to him in a proclamation passed by the Cortes in 1813 that lists him as a loyal supporter of the regency.[4] It seems that Ochoa, who was most likely from a medical background and clearly an appointee of the council rather than of Balmis, was angry with his rank in the expedition. In early November, Balmis wrote to the council that Ochoa was "resentful that the Junta had named Salvany as assistant director."[5] This decision led to sharp disagreements between the two men that left the administration of the undertaking unworkable. Balmis petitioned the council for a solution, and Ochoa was subsequently officially removed in November, only a few weeks before the expedition's departure. Ochoa was not the only source of trouble for the launching of the undertaking. Numerous lawsuits arose from rival shipowners and from lodgings who sought additional compensation from the royal treasury for unpaid bills or in an attempt to profit from the voyage.

The most delicate preparation for the voyage involved the acquisition of children for use as carriers of the vaccine. Balmis had originally proposed using orphans, as they had no immediate family members to seek permission from and could be given a better life in the colonies. This plan leaned heavily on the role of the Church in providing for the care of foundlings as well as on the absolutism of Charles IV, which allowed him to order their purposeful infection and removal across the ocean. While perhaps not as cruel as the linguistic deprivation experiments of Emperor Frederick II in the thirteenth century or the "Monster Study" of Wendell Johnson and Mary Tudor in 1939, the actions of Balmis and Charles would certainly raise ethical concerns today. Considering the fate of many children in foundling hospitals and orphanages, the opportunities offered by the expedition were probably viewed as a godsend. In fact, at the turn of the nineteenth century, the average infant mortality rate for the first year of life at the Santiago de Compostela Royal Hospital Foundling Asylum was 741 per 1000.[6] For those lucky enough to survive past the age of two, adoption was a rare option. Life could be less than promising for orphans in Spain, while removal to the New World presented undreamed-of opportunities.

Orphans presented a unique problem with regard to their medical history, as it could be unknown to the child or the foundling home what ailments or treatments they may have received. Balmis therefore hoped to use very young children because they would have been least likely to have contracted smallpox or been variolated.[7] With royal permission, he wrote to various foundling hospitals and orphanages, requesting that suitable children be sent to him for examination. The expedition's organizer apparently had very specific and strict requirements for participants in the voyage. Church officials in Santiago sent forty-seven boys, of whom only five were deemed suitable. Balmis ultimately selected twenty-two boys—ten from local orphanages, with most coming from La Coruña. The original plan had called for up to twenty-three children, but one of the boys, Camilo Maldonado, was ill and had to be left behind. Maldonado died shortly after Balmis departed, confirming Balmis's decision and exemplifying the high mortality rate among young orphans. The ability to use these orphans as human incubators for the illness represented the extremes of both scientific advancement and absolutism that defined the era.

Along with the children came Isabel Zendal Gómez, the rectoress of the Casa de Expósitos, whose employment was announced by a royal proclamation on October 14, 1803.

The King, in conforming with the proposal of the director of the expedition destined to spread in the Indies the vaccine inoculation, his serene majesty allows that the Rectoress of the House of Foundlings of that city be incorporated in the same expedition as a nurse, with the salary and aid indicated to nurses, so that it takes care during the navigation of the attendance and cleaning of the Children that have to embark and to alleviate the disgust that is experienced in some Parents to trust their children to the care of those, without the relief of a woman of good standing. With this said, I pass the corresponding notice to the Ministry of Finance so that the Rectoress receives in that City the aid of three thousand reales for her habilitation and for the payment in the Indies of the salary of five hundred pesos per year, counted from the day of embarkation and half upon return, which should be the account of the Treasury.[8]

Originally from Galicia, Zendal was also a trained nurse and oversaw the boys in her care as well additional patients. Zendal would go down in Spanish history as a Florence Nightingale–type figure, an early traveling nurse at a time when few if any women participated in the great exploratory undertakings of the era. Interestingly, her own mother had succumbed to smallpox when Zendal was only seven years old.[9] Like many other Spanish children at the time, this would have created an extreme burden on the family, one which Jenner's discovery could have eliminated. Like the Bourbons, she had personal reasons to seek an end to the suffering caused by smallpox. As was all too common for children in her position, Zendal grew up in relative poverty, becoming a single mother at the age of twenty-five. After moving with her child to La Coruña, she eventually rose to become the rectoress of the House of Foundlings. Though later sanitizing attempts sought to portray her only as an ardent young religious figure, Zendal emerges from the archives as a member of a religious order, a single mother, and the first international nurse in history. Her reality is not only more interesting but also praiseworthy for its accomplishments.

CHILDREN OF THE BALMIS EXPEDITION

Name	Age	
Candido	7	
Jacinto	3	
Clemente	6	
Juan Eugenio		Died
Vicente Ferrer	7	
Pasqual Aniceto	3	
Martin	3	
Juan Francisco	9	
Tomas Meliton	3	Died
Juan Antonio	5	Died
Jose Jorge Nicolas de los Dolores	3	
Antonio Veredia	7	
Francisco Antonio	9	
Manuel Maria	3	
Jose Manuel Maria	6	
Domingo Naya	6	
Andres Naya	8	Died
Jose	3	
Vicente Maria Sale y Bellido	3	
Francisco Florencio	5	
Geronimo Maria	7	
Benito Velez[10]	9	

Discounting the missing age of the one child on the list, the average orphan was only 5.47 years old. The decision to use only males was most likely based on a number of factors, including the view that they were more likely than girls to survive the arduous journey, their perceived lack of value in contemporary Spanish society compared with young orphan girls, who could at least be married off, and their lack of employment opportunities in Spain on their maturing.

Balmis's plan called for the boys to be brought to the Americas and used for the purpose of inoculating the local population. After this was accomplished, they were to be educated and housed in the New World at royal expense. Upon reaching adulthood, they would also be secured employment and generally be far better off than if they had remained in Spain. Likewise, the foster parents of the orphans were granted 12–40 reales, with similar awards going to the parents of children who did not pass the initial screening but still chose to send their children for the interview process.[11] This last decision was probably aimed at encouraging participation by families in Spain at a time when Balmis was unsure whether he could fill his quota of orphan children.

In yet another example of his Catholic and Enlightenment thinking, the various race-based caste systems of the American colonies were irrelevant to Balmis in the undertaking of his mission. The vaccine was to be provided to all of Charles's subjects regardless of socioeconomic standing. Likewise, children of any race could be employed as carriers. As Balmis opined, "The accident of color has no adverse influence on the vaccine." Smallpox did not discriminate among socioeconomic levels, and ignoring the poor or Indigenous populations would have left a large reservoir for the virus to continue to thrive in.

While he was slowly putting together the various elements of the expedition, Balmis used his time to begin vaccinating the local population of Spain as well. During the summer and fall of 1803, he traveled extensively around La Coruña and Santiago and throughout Galicia, inoculating thousands. This not only would have provided a larger supply of vaccine material for the journey to America but also would have allowed him and his nurses to perfect their techniques. The irony of vaccinating distant subjects while ignoring those at home was not lost on Charles IV, who soon after Balmis's departure called for a similar push to inoculate all citizens of the Iberian Peninsula.

BALMIS EXPEDITION

With Captain Pedro del Barco y España at the helm, the *María Pita* departed from La Coruña on November 30, 1803. On the same day that local Spanish authorities in New Orleans were officially transferring the territory of Louisiana to Napoleon, who thereafter immediately turned it over to the United States, Madrid was sending forth an expedition to preserve the rest of its empire. The *Gazeta de Madrid* again spoke of the "glorious" expedition and prayed for a speedy crossing to "produce quickly and surely all the good that the King wishes and which awaits humanity."[12] Despite several hundred years of experience traveling the open Atlantic, voyages to the Americas were still fraught with danger. Only three years before, in August of 1800, the US Navy lost two ships—the USS *Insurgent* and USS *Pickering*—from storms in the West Indies. Thus, on the morning of September 5, 1803, Dr. Balmis, not sure he would survive either the trip across the ocean or the trek through the Americas, had his will notarized by Antonio Martínez Llorente in preparation for his voyage.

As the ship left the La Coruña harbor, Balmis immediately inoculated the first four children. While the vaccinations that he had performed around the region over the past few months had produced a considerable quantity of material with which to perform operations, there were still questions about how best to transport it and how long each child would remain a viable carrier. Many of the logistics associated with the voyage were pure conjecture, and the voyage stood as something of an experiment in and of itself. Balmis brought collections of the lymph material in tubes, between glass slides, on pins, threads, and linen, all as part of an experiment to see which remained potent the longest. As for the children, each was cared for immaculately by the doctors and Isabel Zendal. Those who were healthy were supplied with all necessary wants, while those who were infected were carefully watched to harvest the lymph at the appropriate time to prolong its voyage across the ocean.

The first stop for the expedition was to be the Canary Islands. Spanish interest in the archipelago had begun in 1402 with the arrival there of Jean de Béthencourt. The Norman lord set about subjugating the region for the king of Castile, defeating local groups, establishing settlements, and acquiring the rights to land. Various other nobles soon followed, though the Spanish throne did not officially approve of its seizure and incorporation until 1478. It would take a further two decades to finally subdue the Indigenous inhabitants, after which the Canary Islands became a major sugar-growing center for Spain. By the early nineteenth century, sugar production in the Caribbean had largely outpaced that of the Canary Islands, but the area remained a popular waypoint for merchants and explorers such as Humboldt and Balmis.

On December 9, 1803, the *María Pita* landed at the port city of Santa Cruz de Tenerife at 8:00 p.m., after an uneventful nine-day sea voyage from La Coruña. Despite arriving at an unexpected hour, civic authorities moved quickly to begin the process of providing children for inoculation. The following morning, Fernando Cagigal, the Marqués de Casa Cagigal, who was the governor of the islands, called together all the civil and ecclesiastical dignitaries of the domain to his home and praised the expedition. Cagigal remarked that it was their duty "to fight with examples and persuasion the worries of the ignorant."[13] The governor then proceeded with the entire assembly of Canarian elites to the dock of the city, accompanied along the way by music from a military band. The *Gazeta de Madrid* records that Cagigal was the first to embrace one of the orphan boys in his arms and led a parade of them through the capital, complete with artillery salutes. Following the reading of testimonials, ten children of "distinguished families" were vaccinated.[14] Cagigal was an accomplished soldier and Enlightenment author, and his reaction was in keeping with his philosophical beliefs. His grand welcome of the expedition did much to allow for its success in the archipelago and was an example that Balmis hoped to see repeated by leaders and dignitaries in Latin America and the Philippines. Soon the various islands were dispatching boats filled with children to Tenerife for the doctors of the mission to inoculate. As a testament to his success, Balmis requested an additional two thousand copies of

Moreau's treatise on January 6, 1804, having exhausted so many of them in the Canary Islands alone. As originally encouraged by Flores in his initial proposal for the expedition to the council, even the local churches became involved. Parish priest Manuel Díaz, of Santa Cruz de la Palma, preached a sermon shortly after Balmis's arrival, which strongly encouraged parents along religious lines to vaccinate their children.[15]

During his nearly monthlong sojourn on the islands, Balmis heavily engaged himself in educating local medical practitioners and the general public on the process of inoculation. He traveled to various locales in the archipelago, vaccinating in public and explaining the process to all who attended. Finally, the members of the expedition worked with Cagigal to set up a permanent vaccination center at Tenerife to protect future generations as well. This final undertaking became the cornerstone of Balmis's long-term strategy to combat the disease in the Americas and the Philippines.

Though the expedition had started off well in the Canary Islands, it encountered its first stumbling block in Puerto Rico. The Spanish physician had written to the governor of Puerto Rico from the Canary Islands on December 14, 1803, both to keep him informed of the progress of the expedition and to allow him notice to prepare an appropriate arrival for Balmis and the vaccine, in keeping with Flores's original ideas. Both religious and civil pomp and adoration were essential to establish the environment for the public to eagerly accept the operation, and Balmis hoped to ensure this would occur. After departing from the Canary Islands on January 6, the Spanish corvette arrived at Puerto Rico on February 9, 1804, following an eventful crossing of the Atlantic.

In his letters, Balmis recorded that there were fifteen days of storms during the roughly monthlong voyage. One child died during the crossing, and many others were stricken with scurvy.[16] Despite this, Balmis's plan to transport the vaccine using a daisy chain of orphans across the Atlantic Ocean had worked. The vaccine had been carried across over 2,800 nautical miles and arrived safely in the New World. Yet his reception in San Juan proved to be a shadow of the pomp and circumstance that had accompanied his arrival at Tenerife. While Governor Ramón de Castro had dutifully sent a subordinate to receive the expedition members on the dock, the Spanish were hoping for a far grander reception. Balmis quickly discovered that his tepid welcome was not from a lack of resources or foresight but from the fact that the island had already acquired the vaccine.

Francisco Oller y Ferrer, a medical doctor who had been educated in Barcelona before working in various hospitals and royal prisons in Iberia, had been stationed in the Caribbean since 1784. During an outbreak of smallpox in the region in 1792, he not only was responsible for caring for the sick but also for undertaking a massive campaign of variolation to reduce casualties at that time and for the future. It was largely his efforts that resulted in the practice being permitted in Puerto Rico for the first time.[17] Afterward, he apparently kept abreast of the newest developments in inoculation, for when the smallpox outbreak of 1802 struck Puerto Rico, Governor Castro and Dr. Oller moved to acquire vaccine material from Dr. Mondeher of Saint Thomas.

The Danish sugar islands had experienced similar outbreaks as the rest of the Caribbean, largely brought by the arrival of enslaved Africans and European trade ships. An epidemic had struck as recently as the 1780s, causing great loss of life. Around the same time, the Danes began to practice variolation, having most likely acquired the procedure from the British on neighboring Tortola. The subsequent arrival of the Jenner method occurred through two avenues. In February of 1802, the Royal Danish Vaccine Commission launched its own philanthropic expedition, dispatching vaccine material to its few colonies in the New World. Unfortunately, as it was transported in a dried state, it did not survive the journey. A local doctor by the name of John Johnston then took it upon himself to retrieve cowpox matter directly from North America, vaccinating his own children upon his return and establishing its presence on the island.[18] It was from this initial batch that Dr. Oller hoped to gain samples.

In a humanitarian gesture, the Danish governor approved the sending of threads covered in cowpox material in early November. When these failed to arrive in a viable state, Dr. Mondeher sent material encased between glass slides on November 23. Oller managed to vaccinate two of his own sons, both of whom successfully contracted cowpox and survived the procedure. After much debate, Castro and Oller decided to begin a massive vaccination program in December of 1803, only two months before Balmis's arrival. The Danish governor of Saint Thomas helpfully dispatched more material as well as an infected enslaved girl, and civic and religious officials held a ceremony to mark the beginning of the undertaking on the island. Starting with his own two daughters, Castro hurriedly spread the vaccine throughout the capital. Much of the infrastructure and support requested by Balmis, including houses, a central building, and clerical support, were instead granted to Dr. Oller and Dr. Tomás Prieto. By the time the Spanish reached San Juan, Oller had already vaccinated some 1,557 people.[19]

Because of this, Governor Castro's reception was far less enthusiastic than Cagigal's had been. Though the expedition's royal orders included a personal plea from Charles IV that local leaders endeavor to aid in the rapid transmission of the vaccine upon landing, there was no way for Madrid to enforce this request. Still, the town council voted to provide housing for the expedition's crew as well as for the infected children. In addition, Balmis was given an official reception at the governor's mansion, a banquet was thrown in the expedition's honor, and the doctor himself was invited by Castro to attend a dramatic performance that night. Despite this, Balmis was quick to complain about the quality of the lodgings and materials provided to the expedition's members, complaints that Castro tried his best to rectify.[20]

Then, after being informed that vaccination was already well underway, Balmis insisted on organizing his own inoculation event. He reminded Governor Castro that part of his mission called for him to "not only bring vaccine, but to assure its perpetuation." Because of this, he still needed to meet with and instruct all civic and medical leaders.[21] In all, he would host five days of public vaccinations during the month of February. And though

Oller publicly supported the expedition and cared for the sickened José Salvany, Balmis soon turned his anger toward the doctor.

Balmis, perhaps out of professional jealousy or from an honest concern for the quality of the work performed, wrote disparagingly of Dr. Oller and his efforts. Referring to Oller as both incompetent and ineffective, Balmis suggested that Governor Castro had acted more out of a desire to seek fame and royal favor than in hopes of actually halting the epidemic.[22] He spoke of a resident who may have possibly died of smallpox after receiving the vaccine, demanding to see the records of every inoculation performed on the island before his arrival.[23] It is difficult to say what drove Balmis to these ends, though its effect on the local Criollo view of Spain was quite damaging. In a letter to the governor, Balmis openly questioned his competence by writing, "Lacking as Your Lordship is in these lights, it would not be easy to make myself understood."[24] He went on to thank God for the recent death of the aforementioned Dr. Prieto, as it had largely halted the preexisting vaccination efforts. Perhaps most insultingly, he closed his letter by informing Castro that while in the Canary Islands, he, Balmis, had been praised by the Marqués de Casa Cagigal, who wished some artist would "make eternal [his] memory perpetuating the remembrance of [his] commission."[25]

Balmis demanded nothing less than a public announcement that Oller and Castro's efforts had failed and that all those vaccinated needed to be revaccinated in the correct "European method." The governor consulted with the newly appointed bishop, Juan Alejo de Arizmendi. A Puerto Rican native and a proponent of increased public health services, Arizmendi recommended that he himself would volunteer to be revaccinated to set an example for the citizens of the island and to defuse the conflict between the two men. Governor Castro later wrote a manifesto defending himself from subsequent political attacks, laying out what occurred next. When presented with previous patients who had been successfully inoculated by Oller, Balmis flew into a rage, saying, "This seems like a rehearsed episode from a comedy . . . your grace is an ignoramus, a halfwit, go study. . . . Your Grace will be hanged."[26]

Rather than departing immediately though, the Spanish doctor remained on the island for several weeks, hoping to set up a permanent vaccination board as planned in the original mission of the expedition. Apart from simply administering vaccines, these boards would serve several additional purposes. They would help to educate leaders and the local population about the benefit of vaccination. They would encourage the harvest and preservation of cowpox lymph. And they would keep records of all immunizations performed in the region and provide these records to authorities during epidemics. In the event of an outbreak, they would serve as an organizational body.

To avoid a repeat of the situation on the next leg of his journey, Balmis wrote to the civil authorities in Caracas informing them of his immediate departure and laying out his expectations upon arrival. As he prepared to depart in March of 1804, he was again stymied by local officials. The governor was hesitant to approve Balmis's acquisition of children to help spread vaccine material to the continent because of concerns for their safety and future. The council had approved the recruiting of more local orphans or, if these were difficult to find, children with parents, provided Balmis receive approval from both families and local officials. While this would have been a difficult task normally, his behavior while in Puerto Rico rendered it practically unthinkable. Likewise, delays in the expedition's departure and logistical concerns over actually providing the promised money and education in Mexico City created ill will with local parents. In the end, when the ship finally departed for the coast of South America, there were only four boys aboard carrying cowpox material that could be harvested. Without bidding farewell to the governor or council, the expedition members climbed aboard the *María Pita* and prepared to launch. Though the sailing of the vessel was set for March 2, a lack of favorable winds kept it confined to the port for ten days. During this awkward period, city officials continued to feed the members of the expedition, at costs that would eventually reach 2,712 pesos. Despite this continued show of goodwill from the island's government, it was once again not to Balmis's liking.[27]

In the end, the expedition to Puerto Rico was a medical success but a political disaster. Several thousand people were immediately vaccinated through the work of Oller and Balmis, with more to follow over the next few years through the efforts of local civic and medical officials. But several major missteps had occurred. The confrontation between the Spanish physicians and local doctors and leaders can be attributed to a number of factors, including Balmis's own personality, Spanish views of the colonies, and the aforementioned scientific absolutism. Despite his best efforts, Balmis failed to establish a permanent vaccine board to continue his work after he left. Part of this was clearly driven by his contempt for local practitioners, combined with his haste to continue on to the mainland. The professional ill will created during Balmis's brief stay on the island, at a time when popular revolution was threatening around the world, was taken seriously by Charles IV. After receiving letters from Oller and Castro describing Balmis's "shameless actions," the king instructed the newly arrived governor, Toribio Montes, to launch a full investigation of what had occurred. In the end, Montes merely concurred with Oller concerning the efficacy of his previous vaccinations and withdrew himself from the personal fight between the two doctors.[28]

A few days after departing Puerto Rico, the expedition arrived in Puerto Cabello. Not only was the public reception much warmer than it had been in San Juan, but Balmis was presented almost immediately with twenty-eight children to vaccinate, thus ensuring the survival of his lymph material. The delay in departure from San Juan had cost him dearly in terms of time, and as his ship was approaching La Guaira, only one child out of the four aboard was still able to transmit material for inoculation. The warm welcome and quick response of local authorities helped to avert a disastrous end to the expedition.

Unfortunately, tragedy also welcomed Balmis in New Granada, for it was at this stage of the expedition that Balmis learned of the death of Dr. Berges. Berges had been meant to lead the expedition through South America, while Balmis moved through New Spain. Because of this event, as well as the pressing need to take the vaccine farther north, the Spanish physician decided to split the expedition in half to simultaneously deliver cowpox to the various parts of the Spanish colonies.

His assistant director, Dr. José Salvany, was tasked with vaccinating New Granada and points farther south, while Balmis would visit Cuba and New Spain. Once they had acquired enough children and material, Salvany would embark from La Guaira and head to Cartagena. From there he would proceed down the Magdalena River before reaching Santa Fe de Bogotá, and then would proceed onward to Peru and Argentina. His instructions recommended that he acquire two or three children from each locale to use to transport the illness. Likewise, he was encouraged to communicate beforehand with local leaders to ensure a welcoming reception, supplies, and children to use as hosts. Finally, Salvany was asked to make scientific observations of the environment, local arts and industry, and any promising medicines. As well, he was to pay "attention to the specific diseases of each country."[29]

Balmis proceeded from Puerto Cabello toward the city of Caracas, arriving there on April 3, 1804. In a pattern that was becoming more welcome and more familiar, the members of the expedition were greeted with civil fanfare by the population of 42,000.[30] The town council had specifically set aside 80 pesos to welcome and accommodate the expedition, a rather generous sum at the time. After being received by representatives of both the Church and the state, Balmis set out immediately to work. Beginning with two-year-old Luis Blanco, he vaccinated 2,064 children by only his third day in the city. Soon after, at the request of Governor Manuel de Guevara y Vasconcelos, he established a central vaccine board, which was subsequently successful in bringing inoculation throughout the area of northern New Granada and even to some of the islands beyond. By a month's time, some 12,000 people had been protected against smallpox, and by November this number had risen to 38,724.[31]

Balmis departed the city on May 6, 1804, to continue along a prearranged route toward New Spain. His now-reduced band proceeded toward the sea and traveled by boat to Cuba. Arriving on May 27, Balmis discovered that, much like Puerto Rico, the island had already been heavily inoculated. Several months before the expedition's arrival, María Bustamante had sailed there from Puerto Rico, accompanied by her son and two enslaved people.[32] Just prior to their departure, on February 1, a local physician had vaccinated the members of Bustamante's household, allowing them to bring the material to Cuba. In Cuba, Dr. Tomás Romay then harvested the material and used it to vaccinate his own children and hundreds of other residents. Very soon, the practice spread to various parts of Cuba, just as Balmis arrived at Havana.

The Spanish physician, perhaps learning his lesson from Puerto Rico, reacted more positively to the discovery that vaccination was already underway on the island. The governor of the wealthy possession, Salvador José de Muro, second Marquis de Someruelos, received Balmis with as much courtesy and pomp as possible, no doubt contributing to the Spanish doctor's more pleasant demeanor. An official delegation was sent aboard the *María Pita*, and the members of the expedition and the children were dutifully escorted into the city. The carriers of the vaccine were housed with the captain-general, while Balmis was taken to the council and seated in a place of honor.

While on the island, Balmis once again set about creating a local vaccination board that could continue the process of improving public health following his departure. In an interesting attempt to fund its continued operation, he proposed a tax of 2 reales for each enslaved person newly transported to the island. As Cuba was a major transit point for this trade, the move would have raised considerable capital. Ultimately though, colonial officials in Madrid rejected the plan.[33] Finally, Balmis and Dr. Romay undertook a series of experiments on local cows, attempting to infect them with cowpox as a means by which to provide a continuous supply of serum. It is perhaps telling that, in a complete volte-face to what had occurred in San Juan, Balmis worked in conjunction with Romay rather than attempting to subvert the local doctor's efforts. It seems that the Spanish physician soon began to see the treatment as a cure-all for numerous other conditions as well. During his time in Havana, he touted its efficacy against yellow fever, malaria, scabies, and, in keeping with his own previous work in Mexico, venereal disease.[34] In the end, though, this may have been more of an attempt by Balmis to justify his presence on the island as a medical emissary of the king bringing accurate knowledge of the vaccine's true potential, as opposed to local practitioners who had merely stumbled on it.

Having accomplished his task, Balmis departed with much fanfare from Havana on June 18 and reached the port of Sisal, in Yucatán, on June 25. As the dominant political entity in the Spanish colonies in the Americas and with the largest population, New Spain represented the main battleground in the war against smallpox. Balmis's decision to proceed to the area himself clearly demonstrates this. Likewise, Balmis's own history in the region gave him a distinctive knowledge of it, as well as a deep desire to address the health concerns present there. Sickness in Spain affected the trade route from Manila to Madrid that the Spanish Empire still depended on for its economic strength. From Sisal, Balmis proceeded along the road to the regional city of Merida, reaching it on June 28. The captain-general of Yucatán, Benito Pérez Valdelomar, enthusiastically allowed the Spanish physician to vaccinate residents of the city. Sisal and Merida were major ports of entry for Mexico and Guatemala, and the successful vaccination of the residents was vital to the overall public health of the viceroyalty. Interestingly, it was the Spanish foothold in Merida, established in 1542, that had first brought smallpox into the Maya regions of Central America, decimating what remained of that population.

From here, Balmis again split his command, sending his nephew Francisco Pastor south to Guatemala to conduct vaccinations in that region. Pastor departed on July 12, traveling with two vaccinated children by boat to Laguna de Términos. From there he proceeded overland to Villahermosa and Chiapas until he reached Guatemala City in November. The capital had only just been reestablished following its destruction by a series of earthquakes in 1773, thus presenting an interesting sociopolitical environment for the delivery of the vaccine. The new city lacked the entrenched power structures present in Havana and Mexico City, thus reducing resistance to the Spanish expedition. As has been seen, Flores had helped to revolutionize public health in the region during his time in the audiencia, and thus Pastor found a welcoming populace. Yet, the advanced state of medicine in the region also meant that Guatemala had already sought out the vaccine prior to his arrival, and the Spanish physician arrived in the middle of a vast inoculation campaign.

Having failed to garner samples of cowpox lymph from New Orleans and Mexico City, Ignacio Pavón y Muñoz, a native of Guatemala who was living at the time in Mexico, was able to procure some from Veracruz in April of 1804. Most likely, the material he received had originated in Puerto Rico during Balmis's time there. After it was sent to Guatemala, Drs. Narciso Esparragosa y Gallardo and José Antonio de Córdova used it to launch a massive vaccination program. By June 16, a month before Pastor's arrival, civic officials notified Madrid that "thousands of persons of every age, sex, and condition" had been inoculated.[35] By the time Pastor arrived, this number had ballooned to between four thousand and nine thousand.[36] Though the initial attempts by Esparragosa and Córdova in 1802 failed to end the smallpox epidemic then striking the region, the arrival of the Philanthropic Expedition allowed for the accomplishment of their crusade. Though Pastor's presence was perhaps ultimately unnecessary, that of the expedition was not.

As Pastor departed for Central America, Balmis boarded the *María Pita*, and sailed along the Mexican coastline, and reached the port of Veracruz on July 24. It was the major entry point to central Mexico, and the expedition hoped to engage heavily in the city of approximately fifteen thousand before progressing farther inland. Yet the great vaccinator had trouble finding patients to inoculate upon landing, especially young children. Fearing once more that he risked losing his supply of vaccine material, he performed the operation on ten local soldiers instead.

The reason for the lack of interest in his efforts soon became apparent to Balmis. Once again, his own vaccination efforts had outpaced him. José de Iturrigaray had just been appointed to office as the viceroy of New Spain when he decided that "one of the projects that inspired his fervor and desire to please the vassals . . . was to introduce the valuable distribution of the vaccine."[37] Disease and its impact on society and the nation was a perennial concern for leaders in New Spain. As has been seen, it even affected national security, with garrisons in Veracruz experiencing 1,220 deaths from illness from 1799 to 1803 alone.[38] Therefore, with Dr. Alejandro Arboleya, a professor of medicine in Spain who had come over to Mexico with the new viceroy in tow, Iturrigaray acquired samples of the material from Veracruz.[39] These had been brought by the ship *Anfitrite* from Havana, arriving in Mexico weeks before Balmis did. Likewise, Humboldt records that an American, Thomas Murphy, had introduced the vaccine into Mexico City and Morelia even earlier, with perhaps sixty thousand already inoculated by the time of Balmis's landing.[40] This number could be exaggerated, could include cases of variolation, or could have combined figures from Balmis's own efforts later on with earlier ones. Perhaps in an attempt to expound on his own accomplishment and handling of the situation, Governor Iturrigaray also had a copy of the *Gazeta*, which announced the campaign's launch, hand delivered to the Spanish physician while he remained at Veracruz.[41]

This supplement to the *Gazeta*, published on May 26, 1804, contains a firsthand account of the viceroy's efforts. In it he lays out his exhaustive search for viable vaccination material. Lamenting that Balmis's philanthropic expedition had yet to arrive, he proclaims that he was taking it on himself to begin an inoculation campaign, "to please the vassals."[42] Likewise, in yet another attempt to undercut the Spanish mission, Iturrigaray also announced his intent to publish a treatise on the science behind the procedure in order to instruct the various doctors and civil leaders of New Spain on how best to continue what he had started.[43]

Undeterred, Balmis resolved to continue his mission and deliver the vaccine and the orphaned children to Mexico City. Mexico City was the epicenter of the Spanish colonial territories, and Balmis's failure to reach it would perhaps be seen as a failure of the expedition itself. Moving quickly out of Veracruz, he proceeded northwest into the country along the royal highway. By the end of July, he had passed through the region of Xalapa, rapidly moving toward the capital. Part of the reason for his celerity arose from his own fears of contagion. Having spent many years in New Spain, Balmis was well aware of the dangers posed by yellow fever along the coast of Veracruz. As Humboldt had pointed out, "The black vomit finds an insurmountable barrier at the Encero, on the declivity of the mountains of Mexico, in the direction of Xalapa, where oaks begin to appear, and the climate begins to be cool and pleasant, so the yellow fever scarcely ever passes beyond the ridge of mountains."[44] Despite Balmis's best efforts, however, yellow fever did erupt among the members of the expedition, incapacitating many.

After almost two weeks of travel, the medical convoy reached the edge of Mexico City on August 8 and was housed for the night in the small village of Guadalupe, on the outskirts of the capital. Refusing to remain there, however, Balmis and his group proceeded into the city itself, hoping to reach the viceroy's residence. The director's decision to enter the city is puzzling and has been attributed to the poor conditions at Guadalupe or to Balmis's hopes of a triumphant entrance. As the night was well advanced, though, the governor chose to lodge them in a ruined house in one of the poorer districts. Balmis recorded, "We were located at the edge of the slums in the foulest and most feted of them . . . next to a canal in which the city's filth was collected."[45] Balmis clearly saw vitriol in the viceroy's action and choice of housing. Iturrigaray defended his decisions by claiming that the city was unprepared for Balmis's arrival.[46]

Accounts differ as to the motives and actions of Viceroy Iturrigaray, with Balmis frequently arguing for underhanded motives on the part of the royal governor. According to Iturrigaray's own accounts, the viceroy had moved months before to end Balmis's expedition, hoping to gain credit himself as the savior of New Spain.[47] According to Balmis's account, apparently only the intervention of the bishop of Michoacan, Benito María Moxó, allowed Balmis to even land at Veracruz. Some historians have agreed with this view, suggesting a certain level of sabotage on the part of the royal governor.[48] Yet others praise Iturrigaray for his decisive actions, commending him for sponsoring "a great and successful campaign against smallpox . . . countless thousands of his subjects received the treatment free of charge."[49] Still others suggest that Iturrigaray had been personally vaccinated by Balmis as an example to the masses upon the doctor's arrival.[50] Most likely the truth lay somewhere in the middle.

Iturrigaray's largest obstruction to Balmis's mission was his refusal to mandate forced vaccination on the unwilling population.[51] While a firm believer in the procedure, he was opposed to what he saw as an absolutist use of power. Perhaps Balmis had envisioned a repetition of the Canary Islands, where peasants traveled for days and waited in lines for this royal gift. For a variety of reasons, however, the population of central Mexico responded differently. Likewise, the viceroy chose not to follow the proposed guidelines for the establishment of a permanent vaccine board. Instead, after the departure of the expedition, he formed his own structure following consultation with local physicians. Despite this, Balmis had largely achieved his goals: the capital city was being inoculated and local vaccine boards were being established.

Balmis would remain in the city for several weeks, gathering fresh supplies, depositing the orphans in the care of the city, and planning his next moves. Rejoined by his nephew, Francisco Pastor, who had completed his campaign in Central America, the Spanish physician once more decided to split his command in two. Though Iturrigaray had begun vaccinations in Mexico City, he had largely ignored the rest of the province. The sheer vastness of the territory and the large number of towns required a more dispersed method of vaccine distribution. Antonio Gutiérrez Robredo was entrusted with the task of proceeding north to Celaya, Zacatecas, Durango, and Guadalajara, while Balmis moved south to Pueblo, after which both men would rejoin in Acapulco. Balmis not only hoped to provide vaccinations to the locals but also wished to gather more boys for the next leg of his journey, across the Pacific to the Philippines. While Mexico City would normally have been a more appropriate metropolis from which to acquire vaccine carriers, the resistance of the viceroy as well as Balmis's experiences in Puerto Rico perhaps convinced him that he would have to instead scour the countryside for boys.

His initial efforts focused on the town of Puebla. Located to the southeast of Mexico City, it was a major commercial and agricultural hub situated midway between the capital and the Gulf of Mexico. Balmis had written to Manuel de Flon, the mayor of Puebla, both to announce his arrival and to seek Flon's help in spreading inoculation. Perhaps his bout of troubled arrivals upon reaching New Spain had pushed Balmis to seek new solutions on how best to encourage the locals to be vaccinated. In keeping with Balmis's temperament, he seems to have largely blamed the various civic leaders and medical practitioners he encountered for his lack of progress: "The ignorant commoner is only moved by imitation, as you very well know, and needs examples and aids that astonish him before being persuaded."[52] In reply, Flon suggested bypassing civic leaders and engaging church authorities directly. This suggestion was in fact heavily in keeping with the original concepts that Flores had penned for the undertaking. The Spanish crown had legislated in the 1573 and 1681 Laws of the Indies that all citizens should venerate priests as an example to the Native inhabitants. Both Flon and Flores saw this continued practice as key to engaging the Mestizo and Indigenous populations of central Mexico.

Thus in early September, the expedition departed from the capital of the viceroyalty and proceeded southeast on the main route toward Veracruz. Along this route lay the aforementioned important city of Puebla, a region untouched by Iturrigaray's previous attempts at vaccination. In keeping with Flon's idea, on September 20, 1804, Balmis was received by the bishop of the city, Manuel Ignacio González del Campillo. Campillo, a well-respected public figure in the region, had been educated at various seminaries and at the Royal and Pontifical University of Mexico before serving as a lawyer, local governor, and priest.

The close coordination between civil and religious officials in Puebla perfectly reflected traditional Spanish practices regarding public health.[53] The bishop blessed the vaccination caravan and led them in a massive procession into the central square of the city. Once in the cathedral, a mass was offered, with Balmis and the members of the expedition seated in places of honor. Bishop Manuel even led a Te Deum to praise God for the vaccine. Explaining these actions later, Balmis wrote that the bishop sought to receive the inoculation "in such a way as to *entusiasmar* the pueblo." Puebla presents the ideal case of the close coordination among the Church, the state, and science that were the hallmarks of Spanish medical practices and Balmis's own beliefs about what was needed for a successful campaign.

Apart from performing inoculations, of which twelve thousand are reported to have occurred around Puebla from September to November alone, Balmis also set up another vaccination board. To further drive home the religious component of the method to inoculate the general population, he suggested in Article II of the Puebla Vaccine Regulations that the arrival of the vaccine "should be advertised to the public with as many demonstrations of rejoicing and festivity as possible, so that the Indians especially understand that they are being brought a good thing, and that they should present their children to receive it, freeing themselves from the cruel scourge of smallpox." The inclusion of mostly members of the Catholic clergy in the various boards he created further highlights this strategy. For its part, local church leaders seem to have eagerly embraced these plans. The bishop of Antequera in Oaxaca, Antonio Bergosa y Jordán, in fact so fervently supported the practice that he encouraged all priests to administer the inoculation to their parishioners, even offering forty days of indulgence to each recipient.[54]

At the same time, Gutiérrez moved north into the regions of Zacatecas and Nueva Vizcaya (modern-day Durango), mimicking Balmis's actions to the south. These two areas had recently emerged as major mining and cultural centers, and their populations were growing rapidly. Gutiérrez was well received by Francisco Rendón, the intendent of Zacatecas, in November of 1804, who used music, parades, and fireworks to tout the efficacy of the vaccine to the public. The campaign in that city was thereafter largely a success. Several weeks later, though, when Gutiérrez reached Guadalajara, the local mayor, Pedro Catani, was unprepared for his arrival. Gutiérrez was made to wait for several days in the nearby village of San Pedro Tlaquepaque as Catani and the city council readied a grand civil and religious procession. Despite this lack of planning, he was eventually warmly welcomed into the city and driven into the center of Guadalajara in Catani's own official carriage. The usual military parades, Catholic masses, and feasts were subsequently held in his honor.

In fact, the expedition seems to have enjoyed its greatest successes outside of Mexico City. These regions had been outside the focus of previous attempts at vaccination and tended to be staffed by more professional Spanish-born administrators, who had experience in diplomatic endeavors. Gutiérrez had served as Juan de Miralles's personal secretary during his time in the American Revolution and was himself an envoy to the United States in the 1780s. As such, Gutiérrez was undoubtedly aware of American and British efforts to control disease during and after the war, especially in Philadelphia.

By the start of 1805, Balmis had reunited with Gutiérrez at Acapulco and prepared for the next leg of his great journey. Charles IV had authorized bringing the vaccine to his colony in the Philippines, completing his great outreach to the far corners of the Spanish Empire. Balmis recruited more children for an even longer ocean crossing, fitted out a new vessel, and gathered the supplies and equipment he would need to follow in the footsteps of Magellan across the Pacific.

CHAPTER 8

A Return to Cajamarca

But vaccination certainly has been a kind antithesis
to Congreve's rockets,
With which the Doctor paid off an old pox, by borrowing
a new one from an ox.

—LORD BYRON

WHILE BALMIS MOVED NORTH THROUGH the Caribbean and Mexico, his assistant, José Salvany, was tasked with the much more difficult and arduous commission of reaching the far corners of the Spanish Empire in South America. Here geography, weather, and the forces of nature often proved a greater barrier than did recalcitrant Criollo governors and wary peasants. The southern leg of the original expedition covered far more territory than its northern counterpart, with Salvany personally traveling over 4,800 miles from modern-day Venezuela to Bolivia. The landscape varied from open grasslands, to forests, to tropical jungles and traversed both deserts and the indomitable Andes Mountains. Salvany was to be as much an explorer as a doctor.

As Balmis sailed across the Caribbean toward Cuba, Salvany moved westward to Cartagena to begin his assignment. He traveled with three assistants—Manuel Julián Grajales, Rafael Lozano, and Basilio Bolaños—as well as four children, whom he hoped to use as carriers for the vaccine. Chartering the ship *San Luis*, the expedition planned to descend the Magdalena River after first calling at Cartagena, toward the interior of Colombia. The nearly one-thousand-mile-long river begins in the Colombian

Andes and flows northward to the Caribbean Sea. Because of its length and direction, the river had served as a natural artery for trade and communication in the province and would now carry Salvany and his vaccine into the heart of New Granada. Unfortunately, the boat almost immediately foundered on the rocks near the then small village of Barranquilla, at the mouth of the river, on May 13, 1804. "Suffering on those beaches from the severity of the ungrateful climate, hunger, thirst, and nudity, and being cruelly martyred by various insects."[1] Balmis wouldn't hear about the wreck until over a month later on June 17, by which time Salvany was able to repair the damage and continue on toward Cartagena. In the interim, he and his assistants used the time to vaccinate hundreds of locals around the mouth of the river and in the village itself. This resulted both from his general desire to spread the inoculation and from the necessity of acquiring fresh hosts for the vaccine.

Once the boat was repaired, the Spanish proceeded by water and land toward the next major city in the viceroyalty. When they finally reached Cartagena on May 24, they were received with the greatest of fanfare and celebration. In a similar vein to what occurred in parts of Mexico, the team was led in procession into the city and a great mass was held, with a Te Deum sung for the vaccination. Juan Marimón, who was both a priest and a medical doctor, personally led the celebration. Cartagena had grown rapidly to dominate the viceroyalty thanks to its mineral wealth and its safer locale close to Panama. Despite Lord Vernon's failed attack of the port in 1741, a defeat, interestingly, caused more by disease than by Spanish guns, prosperity reigned in the city. By the end of the century, Cartagena had become the dominant urban center of the viceroyalty, with the government largely relocating there from Bogotá.

In keeping with the normal pattern of the expedition, several thousand inoculations were administered and a local board of vaccination was established. The excitement around the expedition is usually highlighted with the story of Alfonso Villavicencio, an aged soldier who offered to become vaccinated and used as a carrier despite already having had smallpox in his youth.² Salvany would write that "all those residents displayed the greatest happiness, and together with the officials they gave repeated thanks to the Almighty . . . for freeing them from the devastating disease in that province."³

The group remained for an extended time in Cartagena because of the various illnesses that they themselves had acquired during their dangerous voyage from Caracas. Salvany's health especially would prove to be one of the most pressing issues and limiting agents on the trek across South America. Apart from the malaria that he had previously contracted and that continued to plague him, the doctor also suffered from tuberculosis, a condition that ultimately led to his demise. While descending the Magdalena, he apparently also contracted an infection that cost him the vision in one of his eyes.⁴

While in the city, the physician undertook to construct a vaccine center, much as Balmis did at his various stops. Beyond this, Salvany also used his time to frequently infect local cattle with cowpox. The various Spanish physicians frequently sought to establish a permanent reservoir for the illness, and the cattle-rich areas of New Spain and New Granada seemed to offer the most opportunity for doing so. Salvany took it on himself to instruct local farmers, officials, and peasants on how to undertake the operations on both people and animals.⁵

After several weeks he gathered ten children from a local orphanage to use as live carriers of the disease for the next leg of his journey. Salvany and his men then finally proceeded down the Magdalena River and into the heart of New Granada. Small villages interspaced the forest along the banks of the river as the Spanish pushed southward. Arriving at the mining town of Tenerife, perched on the banks of the river, the Spanish inoculated several hundred residents before once again proceeding south. Eventually, the forests thinned as the expedition entered the swampy region of the Ciénaga Grande de Santa Marta. From there they moved on to the major town of Santa Cruz de Mompox. The group was received in the city with the now-usual scenes of celebration and worship. "A growing number of people, who with torches lit and bells tolling erupted in acclamations in favor of the expedition's king."[6] A mass followed the entrance parade, and both the monarch and the vaccine were praised. The city was yet another good example of the advanced nature of medicine in the Spanish Empire. A hospital, San Juan de Dios, had been founded in the town in 1550, only twenty-six years after Cortés had organized one in the former Aztec capital, showing the extent to which both medicine and education were emphasized throughout the colonial empire. Here the doctors of the expedition not only inoculated civilians but, once again, the many cows of the region. With the vast Los Llanos region of tropical grasslands stretching from Colombia to Venezuela along the Orinoco and Meta Rivers, cattle ranching was a major source of the income of New Granada and a potential host of domestic supplies of cowpox. As did Balmis, Salvany hoped to establish a permanent presence for cowpox in the region to use for future generations.

After leaving Mompox, the expedition again split. Half continued down the Magdalena River valley toward Santa Fe de Bogotá, while the other group moved into the Ocaña region and Cúcuta Valley. The city of Honda, which served as the main river port for Bogotá farther up the Magdalena, was specifically targeted. Some two thousand vaccinations were performed in Honda.[7] Amidst the region, which would witness the pivotal battles of Simón Bolívar's campaigns only eight years later, the Spanish crown saved the lives of thousands. Salvany recorded that his team vaccinated around fifty-seven thousand people between Cartagena and Bogotá.[8] The two groups soon united once more, and several months later entered into Bogotá on December 17, 1804.

Smallpox had long been associated with the city. Contemporaneous sources record that an outbreak of the disease occurred in 1587 and burned across the region for two years. It is claimed that 90 percent of the Indigenous people who lived in Bogotá at that time succumbed to the disease.[9] Though the exact number of deaths attributed to the pestilence is debatable, its frequent devastating attacks on the capital are not. Like all other major cities in the region, Bogotá was periodically held captive by the disease.

What followed in the capital of New Granada was yet another grand reception by civic and church leaders. Antonio José Amar y Borbón, the new viceroy of New Granada, had only arrived in the territory in September and was eager to carry out Charles IV's orders as well as place his administration on a secure footing. His predecessor, Pedro Mendinueta, though highly successful in organizing the region's response to the smallpox epidemic, had been unable to procure vaccines from other parts of the Western Hemisphere or find a local source from which to extract material. To Amar, the expedition provided a means by which to accomplish his goals. Salvany and his men were feted by the elite of the capital and quickly found a steady source of patients. Andrés María Rosillo y Meruelo, a highly respected local priest, gave a sermon in the city's main cathedral on February 24, 1805, praising Charles IV and the members of the expedition. Rosillo, a native of Socorro, had spent much of his life working to improve medical care in the region, having previously been the president of Del Rosario University.

The sermon, which was later recorded and subsequently published, was built around the notion of punishment and redemption. Both the disease and its cure were to be seen as proof of God's divine plan. Beginning with a reference to Isaiah 63:4, "It was for me the day of vengeance; the year for me to redeem had come," Father Rosillo lends all credit to God for "redeeming us from the plague."[10] The history of the disease is recounted from its assumed arrival in Spain in the seventh century to the destruction it now visited periodically on the world. Rosillo goes on to praise "the immortal Edward Jenner, [who] tore apart that hydra" and who served as the instrument of God in the creation of the vaccine. King Charles is then praised as having had the care and ability to organize the expedition to save his people and provide them with "a redemption of health and life." Interestingly, though, neither Balmis nor Salvany are mentioned in the sermon. Perhaps their absence arose from a desire to focus on the divine author of the expedition, or perhaps it once more showed the local disdain toward the visiting doctors.

Despite this minor oversight, the small group undertook the initial vaccination of two thousand residents following their grand reception. Salvany held eight such sessions, each of which was aimed at both inoculating locals and instructing priests and doctors how best to carry out the procedure in the future. In keeping with the goals of the expedition, Salvany also established a central board of vaccination before he ultimately departed from Bogotá. One of Salvany's more interesting receptions within the city was with José Celestino Mutis. The famed Spanish botanist was currently in Santa Fe de Bogotá continuing his research and took it on himself to meet with the medical team to praise and encourage the continuation of their work.[11]

Despite Salvany's tuberculosis worsening to the point that he was frequently expelling blood from his lungs, he was determined to complete the mission. Geography was beginning to become a far greater enemy to the Spanish physician than his own health was. Lands to the north, east, and south clamored for the cure, and Salvany lacked the ability and manpower to reach every locale. One of these places was Portobelo, in modern-day Panama. Apart from Sir Francis Drake's death in the region from dysentery, numerous outbreaks of yellow fever and malaria, and several attacks by the English over the previous century, smallpox was also a reoccurring problem. A local legend and cult even arose around the image of the Black Christ of Portobelo. According to tradition, the statue arrived in a box that floated into the harbor during an outbreak of smallpox in 1658. Once it was removed from the container and venerated in the Church of San Felipe, the epidemic ended.[12] Because of the town's importance as the center point of the Asia-America-Spain trade network, the vaccine was sent there for local doctors to administer. This saved Salvany and his men a lengthy diversion following their departure from Cartagena yet still allowed for the vaccine to reach this important population center.

In order to cover more territory in the rapidly expanding geography of South America, Salvany and his men again split into two teams in February of 1805, following their success at Bogotá. One group passed over the

Cordillera Occidental and proceeded through the Chocó region, Ibagué, and Ibarra to reach Quito. The second group followed the eastern side of the mountains, vaccinating La Plata and Pasto before entering Quito from the east. After rejoining in the future capital of Ecuador, one group was to proceed to Guayaquil and then move south into Chile while Salvany moved into Peru. It was a slow progression through forests and over mountain chains, further hindered, no doubt, by the doctor's declining health. It would take until December of 1805 for both groups to reach Quito.

Once again, the Spanish physicians and children received a welcoming reception. Quito had been troubled by smallpox as frequently as other major cities in the region had, losing over one-third of its population to the disease in 1589. Unfortunately, Salvany's health continued to falter, and the group was forced to wait in Quito for two months while he slowly recovered his strength.[13] The members of the expedition were by no means idle during this time. Thousands were inoculated and another vaccine board was established to cover the region along the Pacific coast.

Despite its isolation in terms both of elevation in the mountains and distance from other major locales, the city had a long history of medical exploration. The founding of the Universidad Pontificia De San Gregorio Magno in the early seventeenth century, though well after the construction of similar institutions in Mexico City, Bogotá, and Lima, allowed for the training of doctors and the advancement of science in the region. Two notable physicians from the region, Juan Bautista Aguirre and Eugenio Espejo, did much of their work with microbes and smallpox. Espejo, specifically, theorized a connection between microscopic life and the transmission of the disease: "Within the infinite variety of these living particles we have an admirable resource to explain the prodigious multitude of diseases and symptoms."[14] Salvany once again found fertile ground in the medical and academic circles of Quito.

This trend continued in the immediate outskirts of the city as well, as the Spanish moved southward toward Guayaquil and Peru. In the important town of Cuenca, located over four hundred kilometers to the south, the

Spanish were again celebrated and feted by the locals. A series of bullfights and a masquerade were held to honor the expedition's arrival, and the local churches were officially illuminated for three nights in a gesture of thanksgiving. A few weeks later, Salvany was further celebrated in the town of Loja, where he undertook 1,500 vaccinations and again sought to infect the local bovine population.

Not all villages and towns reacted so positively to Salvany's arrival. As the expedition wound its way deeper into the continent, it began to be confronted by more Indigenous villages. These tended to be more isolated, traditional, and untouched by either regional administration or dictates from Spain. While Salvany continued to vaccinate thousands, he acknowledged in his letters and reports the more cautious attitude of the Indigenous people toward the practice, an attitude that sometimes bordered on anger and violence. In the small village of Chocope, the physician wrote that "the Indians are, with certain justice, accustomed to doubt everything proposed to them by the white man."[15] Apparently, after seeing the ease with which the operation was performed, an operation that would ostensibly wipe out the greatest killer of their ancestors, the Native inhabitants became angry at Salvany, doubting his efforts. Only the intercession of a local village priest managed to save his life. Similar scenes unfolded in several other Native towns.

Salvany grew concerned about the state of sanitation in local hospitals. These generally served as the focus point for all efforts to inoculate, yet less than ideal conditions could lead to any number of epidemiological problems. "The noxious airs one breathes in the hospitals can alter and discredit the vaccine."[16] Though his reasoning may have been flawed, there certainly was a legitimate health concern for those entering these facilities. To remedy this, Salvany proposed the creation of chapter houses that would focus solely on the dispersal of vaccine material, thus reducing the number of healthy people entering hospitals and also conserving hospitals' resources.

Despite his large successes up to this date, his expedition's movement and actions into the interior of New Granada soon began to be outpaced by the natural trade in materials along the Pacific coast. In a similar pattern to what occurred in Mexico City, Salvany heard as he moved southward that inoculations were already being carried out in Lima. The viceroy, Gabriel de Avilés, had dispatched Dr. Pedro Belomo to Buenos Aires to acquire samples of the vaccine. Once there, Belomo most likely received it from Dr. Miguel O'Gorman, who had only recently acquired the material himself from London via the Portuguese. Returning in October of 1805 and using enslaved Africans as carriers, Belomo proceeded to offer inoculation to the inhabitants of the capital but experienced much resistance. Despite monetary compensation from the governor, the population was hesitant, and in the end Belomo managed to vaccinate only around three dozen people before his supply chain ended.

Avilés, like many other Spanish leaders of the time, was eager to address the public health issues of his province. After helping to put down the uprising of Túpac Amaru II in the 1780s, Avilés slowly rose through the ranks of colonial administration. While governor of Chile, he opened hospitals, reformed medical education in the region, and worked to improve public safety and sanitation. Though he began the official search for vaccine material in the region, large-scale inoculation would occur after the inauguration of his successor, José Fernando de Abascal y Sousa.

Salvany sought to rapidly move along the Pacific coast of Peru and reach Lima, but his health and local affairs stood in his way. Perhaps he was driven by his own looming demise or a desire to seize control of the vaccination operation then in progress in the capital, or perhaps he simply wanted to proceed to farther provinces. After leaving Piura, he heard of an outbreak of smallpox in Trujillo and quickly moved to combat it through the use of his vaccine material. Along the journey, his health worsened and a mutiny broke out among his native porters. Salvany was forced to seek shelter in the small village of Paysandú, whose locals were quite eager to be inoculated. Their actions helped to preserve the material and allowed for the continuation of the journey to the south.

Despite successfully defeating the outbreak of smallpox in Trujillo, the Spaniards faced disease, rebellion, and political resistance as they moved through the northern half of Peru. Local leaders in the town of Lambayeque, epitomizing these difficulties, refused to grant Salvany and his men a reception upon their arrival. Salvany's worsening tuberculosis seems to have unnerved his local porters and guides, who frequently abandoned him.[17] The expedition's members struggled through the rough hinterlands of Peru until a local resident found them and helped conduct them to the mining town of Chota. Here they rested, inoculated residents, and trained local practitioners before proceeding toward Lima. The nadir of this leg of the journey came during Salvany's return to Trujillo a few months after his initial success in defeating the smallpox outbreak there. Local opposition to and lack of interest in vaccination reached such a level that Salvany resorted to forced vaccination simply to preserve his supply of cowpox material.[18]

Six months after entering Peru, in March of 1806, Salvany finally reached Cajamarca. The town that had witnessed thousands killed during the initial Spanish conquest of the Inca in 1532 now saw thousands saved by the power of European medical technology. Yet the hostility that Salvany had begun to witness in northern Peru continued as he moved deeper into the country. He frequently recorded his frustration at the lack of medical services and experts in the interior of the Spanish Empire as well as at the behavior of the Indigenous populations.[19] Native people in Ica began to spread rumors that the expedition was there to kidnap children, leading to widespread panic and the exodus of families to the mountains as Salvany approached.[20] Cajamarca, as a major town, was one of the few exceptions to the trend of poorly organized reception and medical services that the expedition increasingly encountered in the region of Peru. The leader of Cajamarca, Joaquín Miguel de Arnaco, dutifully organized the type of civil and religious reception that Salvany had become accustomed to in New Granada.

Two months later, on May 23, 1806, an exhausted and illness-stricken Salvany arrived in the colonial capital, Lima. Since viable vaccinations had already been procured from Argentina, the process had become a profitable one in the capital, so many of the local doctors and merchants reacted harshly to the royal expedition's arrival. Though his initial reception was poor, Salvany was eventually warmly welcomed following the arrival of the new viceroy. In August of 1806, José Fernando de Abascal took office in Peru. A promoter of educational reform and public health improvement, Abascal eagerly embraced Salvany and his mission. By October, Salvany reported performing twenty-two thousand inoculations, a total that represented perhaps one-third of the population at the time. Professor Hipólito Unanue, who did much to expand the medical education of the city and province during the early nineteenth century, personally eulogized Salvany to the University of San Marcos and presented him with an honorary degree. His statement, "And you, kind Salvany, that by obeying the orders of such a great King, you have exposed yourself to so many dangers by sea and land, enter to rest from them, occupying a seat among the enlightened Doctors of this University," in many ways fails to express the actual magnitude of Salvany's accomplishments.

Yet tensions continued below the surface. Many considered Salvany an outsider and resented the scientific imperialism that accompanied his arrival. At the same time, local practitioners stood to lose business in the face of gratuitous inoculation by the Bourbon dynasty. By September of 1806, while Salvany was being lauded at the University of San Marcos, the city council actively discussed replacing him with Pedro Belomo as the coordinator of the vaccine board. A feud soon developed between the two men, which Salvany ultimately lost.[21] Even Unanue's speech delivered during the award of Salvany's honorary degree lauded "the cow, the inestimable animal," nearly as much as it did the Spanish doctor.[22] Local doctors even began to claim that it was their own efforts that had inspired the crown to dispatch the expedition in the first place, assertions that Salvany sought to publicly denounce. For many in Lima, this was also Spain's effort to assert their presence on a continent dominated politically by Bogotá and New Granada.[23] By the start of the year

1807, the expedition's mission in Lima had largely been subsumed by local officials.

Despite these confrontations, when the expedition departed from the capital in January of 1807, some 197,000 people had been vaccinated in the viceroyalty. With two inoculated children in tow, the group headed southeast along the western side of the Andes, deeper into the Spanish Empire. The group again split at this point, with Grajales and Bolaños assigned to move east toward the Andes. Their bailiwick would include the towns of Huarochirí, Jauja, Tarma, and Canta, before departing for Chile. At the same time, Lozano moved toward Ayacucho and the ancient Inca seat at Cuzco.

Salvany was once again beset by health issues and troubles with his porters. His worsening tuberculosis caused his drivers to abandon him in February of 1807 as he neared the town of Chinca. After several weeks of recovery, he continued his journey, and finally reached Ica in April. Though the number of vaccinations he was able to deliver had grown rapidly since his departure from Lima, he once again was confronted by mistrust and rumor in the town of Ica. In the end, Salvany would inoculate only some 352 individuals, a small fraction of the population. After several unsuccessful weeks, he continued his journey, reaching Nazca on July 30. Here the receptions began to improve for the members of the expedition, with hundreds of inoculations performed in Nazca, Acarí, Camaná, and Arequipa. At the last of these towns, a public reception was held and a Te Deum proclaimed at the local church, harkening back to previous such welcomes in New Granada. The acclaim that Salvany received in Arequipa proved timely, as his tuberculosis reached its final stage.

Salvany was forced to stay in the town of Arequipa for a year, slowly gathering his strength. While small vaccinating teams were dispatched to neighboring villages, this leg of the expedition largely came to a standstill. It would take until the late summer of 1808 for him to depart again. By September, he had reached the town of Puno, on the shores of Lake Titicaca. The group was again forced to halt because of Salvany's illness, this time a minor heart ailment. His rapidly declining health was severely affecting the speed and success of the expedition. Despite this, he was well received and the vaccine was administered to the public. The letters written afterward by the civic leaders of the town to Charles IV highlight one of the principal concerns of colonial administrators regarding smallpox. After thanking the monarch for sending the vaccine to the Americas, they noted that it would allow them to conquer smallpox and ensure a larger Indigenous workforce for the mines of the region.[24]

After recovering his health sufficiently, Salvany continued to skirt the southern boundary of the lake, slowly crossing the scrub grasslands of the Peru-Bolivia border. In March of 1809, the group entered the town of La Paz. Salvany's earlier rapid progress through New Granada had slowed to a crawl in the Andean region of South America. He was so weak by this point that he wrote to Lima and Cádiz asking to be replaced so that the inoculation campaign could continue at a much quicker pace without him restraining it.[25] No replacement was granted. Finally, on July 21, 1810, Dr. José Salvany succumbed to tuberculosis in Cochabamba, Bolivia. A public funeral was held for him, and his remains were committed to a now-forgotten tomb in the Church of San Francisco in Cochabamba.

The various auxiliary inoculation teams dispatched by Salvany continued their work after his death. Grajales and his assistant vaccinated around ten thousand individuals in the mountains of Peru and continued through Chile and Argentina, not ending their expedition until 1812. At the same time, Lozano focused on the region of Cuzco, where he performed around twenty-four thousand inoculations. Grajales took to the ocean to continue his trek down the western edge of South America, rather than going overland from Peru. Considering the ongoing naval war with the United Kingdom at the time, this was a far more dangerous voyage than continuing through the Andes. Despite the risk, however, his small group made it safely to Valparaíso in December of 1807. Grajales immediately undertook the vaccination of over eight hundred people, and in January of 1808, he established a board of vaccinations to continue the efforts upon his departure.[26]

Grajales visited several towns in the northern part of Chile, including Quillota, Aconcagua, Casablanca, and Melipilla. Continuing to the east, he finally arrived in Santiago in April of 1808. Ambrosio O'Higgins Road, which connected the two cities of Santiago and Melipilla, had only recently been completed, allowing for movement of more trade, communication, and, in this case, medical aid between Santiago and the coast. Though the local governor, Luis Muñoz de Gúzman, had died two months before, Grajales found a welcoming replacement in Francisco Antonio García Carrasco. The new governor provided the official and material support necessary to make the inoculation campaign in the capital a notable success.[27] Over eight thousand people were vaccinated in the capital over the course of the next few months, and another vaccination board was established. Grajales remained in the town for over six months, not departing until January of 1809. He most likely spent this time inoculating the inhabitants as well as helping to improve on existing medical services in the far reaches of the Spanish Empire.

Over the course of the next two years, Grajales journeyed through Talca and Concepción and finally reached Valdivia in September of 1810. The extreme southern region of South America was still only sparsely settled by the Spanish, being largely inhabited by the Mapuche people. In keeping with its original philosophy, the expedition drew no distinction between the Spanish inhabitants of the region and the Indigenous people, inoculating both groups. In 1811, Grajales proceeded by boat to Chiloé Island and other parts of the Chilean archipelago, as far south as the forty-eighth parallel. These regions had been ravaged by a smallpox outbreak in 1562 that had decimated the Native population. Despite this, Spanish settlement was sparse and constantly threatened by European raids and Native attacks. As rebellion was already engulfing the region of Chile, Grajales decided to return to Lima in January of 1812, having covered five thousand leagues by land and ten thousand by sea.[28]

Between Balmis, Salvany, and their various adjuncts, Jenner's smallpox vaccination covered the land from Durango in the north to Chile in the south. Tens of thousands of miles had been crossed and hundreds of thousands of imperial subjects inoculated. Race, class, caste, socioeconomic level, and geographic constraints were ignored by Charles IV, Balmis, and Salvany in an expedition that highlighted the most glorious elements of the Enlightenment and the Scientific Revolution.

Balmis in Asia and After

Unlike the mediocre, intrepid spirits seek victory over those
things that seem impossible. . . . It is with an iron will that
they embark on the most daring of all endeavors.
—FERDINAND MAGELLAN

IN SEPTEMBER OF 1519, the Portuguese explorer Ferdinand Magellan departed from Sanlúcar de Barrameda with five ships and 270 men. His mission was to circumnavigate the planet and achieve Columbus's original dream of demonstrating the feasibility of reaching Asia by sea. The Spice Islands of Indonesia and the markets of China had always been the ultimate goal in the European race to explore the world, and recent geographic discoveries led Magellan and others to believe that there still must be some way to sail around the Americas and reach Asia. By November of 1520, Magellan had managed to discover a passage between Chile and Tierra del Fuego and finally had reached the great Pacific Ocean. Mutiny, disasters, and disease stalked his ships as they ventured to the East Indies, despite Magellan's optimism. Finally, on March 16, 1521, the Spanish made landfall in the Philippines. Though the great explorer was killed by the inhabitants of Mactan Island, off of Cebu, his remaining men were able to return to Spain by September of 1522. Nearly three hundred years after Magellan landed in the Philippines, another great Spanish expedition followed a similar route, arriving in a very changed Asia and bringing not trade or conquest but a medical marvel.

It would take almost forty years after Magellan's arrival in 1521 for the

Spanish to begin establishing small settlements on the islands and sub-jugating the local tribes and kingdoms. Though a pattern of colonization similar to that of the Americas developed in the Philippines, because of the unique geography of the islands and their distance from Spain, smallpox arrived there much later than it did in the other Spanish colonies. While the Philippines's close proximity to the Asian mainland would suggest previous arrivals of the pestilence from China or Japan, the limited population of the island chain and its low population density would have restricted its impact. The first recorded outbreak in the post–Magellan era seems to have occurred in 1574, possibly transported by soldiers or merchants, a few years after the first concentrated attempt by the Spanish to secure the region. The Augustinian missionary Martín de Rada, who originally accompanied the Spanish fleet there in 1565, wrote, "A general epidemic of smallpox has raged here since this year, which has spared neither childhood, youth, nor old age; I believe there are few who have not had it . . . and many have died of it."[1]

Smallpox would thereafter descend on the Philippines in periodic waves in a similar fashion as it did in the rest of the Spanish colonial empire. The disease arrived with Spanish soldiers, merchants, and settlers and was carried over from China by trade during the seventeenth and eighteenth centuries. Spanish military operations caused outbreaks in Cagayan Province in the 1600s, in Bohol in the 1750s, and in Samar and Leyte in the 1760s. The last outbreak proved to be particularly devastating, killing an estimated one-third of the population. In 1789, an outbreak from China spread to the Ilocos region, decimating the population there. Spanish efforts to unite the region and improve transportation, communication, and trade probably worsened these outbreaks, as disease could move quickly among formally isolated tribes. Therefore, by 1800, smallpox was as large a threat to the socioeconomic well-being of the Philippines as it was to other Spanish possessions.

Francisco Balmis spent months organizing the final leg of his expedition while in Mexico, before leaving in February of 1805. He acquired twenty-six children, many of whom came from families, to use as live carriers across the Pacific Ocean. Unlike the children brought over the Atlantic, these children were to be returned to New Spain upon completion of the mission. This resulted from their not being orphans as well as from the view that Mexico was a much more desirable colony to live in than the Philippines were. During the weeks spent finding proper vaccine carriers, it soon became evident that volunteers were not as abundant as they had been in Spain. This was due to the nature of the crossing and a lack of support from the viceroy of New Spain. Unlike in Spain, where royal approval led to enthusiastic recruiting, officials in Mexico either failed to support Balmis or actively opposed him. Thus the Spanish were forced to resort to monetary gifts, church influence, and royal prestige to acquire the children. Balmis later wrote disparagingly of the Indigenous subjects of Mexico, who "esteemed more a pecuniary gratification than the great reward that the king offered to keep them and their children later until the age [of maturity], accommodating them."[2] In the end, after much effort, the expedition was able to acquire enough live carriers to transport the vaccine material across the Pacific Ocean. Overseeing the children was Isabel Zendal Gómez, who despite having fulfilled her original contract, chose to remain with Balmis for the Pacific crossing. The children were provided with all the necessities for travel, including matching outfits with jackets emblazoned with a crest that read "I serve the Serene Queen of Asturias."

Balmis's inclusion of children from several major social groups in Mexico is interesting and points to his previous comments on the disease and vaccine knowing no racial boundaries, as well as perhaps to his trouble in finding willing participants.

Spanish trade and communication with Asia remained a difficult and rare event, despite several centuries having passed since Magellan's efforts.

Only once in every year did a single ship, the Nao de la China, sail from Acapulco, on the Mexican shore of the Pacific, slowly traverse

CHILDREN TRANSPORTED ACROSS THE PACIFIC

Name	Town	Age	Race
Juan Nepomuceno Torrescano	Valladolid	6	Spanish
Juan Josef Santa Maria	Valladolid	5	Spanish
Josef Antonio Marmolejo	Valladolid	5	Spanish
Josef Silverio Ortiz	Valladolid	5	Spanish
Laureano Reyes	Valladolid	6	Spanish
Jose Maria Lorechaga	Valladolid	5	Spanish
Josef Agapito Yilan	Guadalajara	5	Spanish
Josef Feliciano Gomez	Guadalajara	6	Spanish
Josef Lino Velazquez	Guadalajara	5	Spanish
Josef Mauricio Macias	Guadalajara	5	Mestizo
Jose Ignacio Najera	Guadalajara	5	Indian
Jose Maria Ursula	Querétaro	5	Indian
Teofilo Romero	Zacatecas	6	Spanish
Felix Barraza	Zacatecas	5	Spanish
Josef Mariano Portillo	Zacatecas	6	Spanish
Martin Marques	Zacatecas	4	Spanish
Josef Antonio Salazar	Zacatecas	5	Mestizo
Pedro Nolasco Mesa	Zacatecas	5	Mestizo
Josef Castillo Moreno	Fresnillo		Spanish
Juan Amador Castaneda	Fresnillo	6	Mestizo
Josef Felipe Osorio Moreno	Fresnillo	6	Spanish
Josef Francisco	Fresnillo	6	Spanish
Josef Catalino Rivera	Fresnillo	6	Spanish
Buenaventura Safiro	Bonnet	4	Spanish
Josef Teodoro Olivas	Bonnet	5	Mestizo
Guillermo Toledo Pino	León	5	Spanish

the great ocean spaces, and discharge at Manila her cargo of arms, munitions, cultural appliances, seeds and woollen stuffs; also she brought there the several months' old mail from America and Spain, along with some officials, soldiers or missionaries. Then she set off on her return voyage to Mexico, loaded with silk and Chinese porcelains, spices and camphor, and having on board an occasional Spaniard who, having sailed the breadth of the Pacific, crossed on muleback the desert plateaux of Mexico, and scudded before the Atlantic storms, might at long last, sometimes in a matter of years, see again his native land.[3]

At the same time, the escalation of the War of the Third Coalition was beginning to affect New Spain. Madrid's role in the conflict, while of secondary importance to that of Paris's role, still required money and resources, all of which began to be drained from the colonies in the Americas. José de Iturrigaray was required to implement new taxation policies that proved to be very unpopular with the people, as was his favorable treatment toward certain social classes. Overall, New Spain had little to spare to assist Balmis's trip across the Pacific, nor was there much interest in sacrificing population and resources to help the Philippines.

The journey from Acapulco toward Asia undertaken in the late winter of 1805, while calm in terms of weather, saw a violent confrontation between the Spanish doctor and the ship's captain. Balmis had chartered the fittingly named *Magallanes* from Angel Crespo for use in reaching the Philippines. Crespo charged an excessive fee of 11,300 pesos for the crossing, demanding 300 pesos for each child and 500 for each adult, a far cry from the 200 normally charged for passengers.[4] On top of these high rates, the ship was overbooked for the crossing because of the rarity of exchange with Asia, having already taken aboard 77 priests and 54 soldiers.[5] Packed aboard a vessel with over 390 persons, the children were relegated to being kept "in a magazine full of filth and large rats."[6] The presence of so much gunpowder in close proximity to the vaccine carriers meant that lamps and open flames would have been forbidden, thus most of the voyage would have been spent in dark and filthy sur-roundings. Worse though, the close proximity of the boys meant that the virus spread more rapidly among them then had been planned, seriously jeopardizing the entire undertaking.[7] A furious Balmis complained to the governor-general of the Philippines upon landing, demanding that the ship's owner be punished. When little action was taken, relations between the two men quickly soured.

Interestingly, the voyage across the Pacific seems not to have involved calling at the Spanish Mariana Islands. Initially claimed in the sixteenth century, serious colonization and conquest of the region did not begin until the second half of the seventeenth century. Despite this, the islands were a routine port for ships voyaging across the ocean, including the Malaspina Expedition of a decade before. As with most other territories of the region, disease had affected the island greatly. Following the mission of Father Diego Luis de San Vitores to the island of Guam in 1668, small-pox became a regular visitor to the area. By the mid-nineteenth century, the population of the major island had fallen from a seventeenth-century high of 40,000 to around 8,207 people. The arrival of smallpox aboard the American merchant ship *Frost* in 1856 brought this number down to only 3,644.[8] Perhaps because of the desire to quickly proceed to Manila or because of opposition from the ship's captain, no concerted effort was made to land on Guam or to vaccinate the local population on the various Spanish Pacific islands.

Rafael María de Aguilar y Ponce de León had been the governor-gen-eral of the Philippines since 1793. During this time, he had done much to upgrade the defenses of the islands as well as to better the archipelago's infrastructure. In fact, the ongoing Napoleonic Wars and concurrent Brit-ish attempts to expand in the Pacific were understandably far more imme-diately pressing matters to Aguilar than the health of his subjects was. Most notably, as recently as 1798, a British warship under the command of Edward Cooke had managed to penetrate the harbor at Manila and capture three gunboats and numerous Spanish sailors and officers. As with many of the other royal appointees of Charles III and Charles IV, Aguilar was a product of the Enlightenment. Therefore, outside of the current and pressing issues of territorial defense, he was a staunch supporter of free trade and the improvement of public health in his colony.

In fact, the governor proved to be an ardent proponent of the process of vaccination, though he was cooler to the person of Balmis, an increasingly common occurrence over the course of the expedition. Tension between Aguilar and Balmis resulted from the latter's insistence on an immediate resolution to his conflict with Crespo as well as from his disgruntlement at being delayed the proper welcome he demanded. While the arrival of the *Magallanes* on Easter Sunday would have clearly affected the organization of a welcoming reception, Aguilar also failed to respond to repeated letters from Balmis for the next several days. Despite this, the governor was generally interested in the process of inoculation. Following the expedition's arrival at Manila on April 15, 1805, an event marked by a flotilla of local ships that welcomed the *Magallanes*, Aguilar promptly had his own five children inoculated as an example to the population.[9] Likewise, following Balmis's departure, Aguilar set up a central vaccine board, of which he himself was president.[10] It was the archbishop of the metropolis who proved to be a far greater initial hindrance to the operation. Juan Antonio Zulaibar, OP, proved to be rather unreceptive to the process and did not provide the grand religious reception that the Spanish doctors had received in the Americas. Zulaibar's opposition is puzzling, though the fact that he had been appointed to the position only several months before and would not be officially ordained until July of 1805 may have played a role. Likewise, legitimate concern did exist as to the effectiveness of the vaccine after its long ocean voyage. This perhaps is what compelled Aguilar to have his own children vaccinated first before raising the hopes of the local population.[11]

Having seen the results in his own children and having read Balmis's treatise on the past successes of the expedition in the Americas, Aguilar soon moved to throw the entire weight of his office behind the program.

The treatment that you may consider convenient to help those villages administered by clergymen in order to convince their inhabitants to accept the vaccination that will preserve them from the destructive and terrible plague called natural smallpox by means of a very simple method in order to defend their children from such a dreadful disease which most of the time leads victims to death and in cases of survival to remain forever full of defects.[12]

Likewise, Balmis soon found support from Francisco Diaz Durana, the dean of the Manila Cathedral. Eventually, after carefully studying the Spanish doctor's work, Fr. Zulaibar came around and was an ardent supporter of the process. In a memorandum sent to church officials in the region on May 29, 1805, Zulaibar recommended measures similar to those undertaken by the Church in Latin America, including the instruction of priests on the benefits of the process and the preaching of the method to parishioners.[13]

Following this, Balmis quickly set to work. By the middle of May, he had already vaccinated several thousand persons and had set up a distribution center for future efforts. Because of the geography of the region, specifically the massive number of islands that made up the archipelago, the expedition was soon forced to split its efforts. While Antonio Gutiérrez Robredo worked in Manila, Santa Cruz, and Cebu, Antonio Pastor and Pedro Ortega traveled to the regions of Zamboanga and Mindanao. Luckily, the short distance between the major islands meant that live carriers would be unnecessary. The material itself was instead shipped in glycerin, between two glass slides, and sealed in wax. As in the Americas, Balmis also established a vaccine center in Manila, which he hoped would continue his work after his departure. The calves of the native water buffalo, known as carabao, proved particularly useful for producing more of the cowpox material needed to carry out subsequent vaccine campaigns as the nineteenth century progressed.[14]

Like the more Indigenous populations of South America, the Filipino population generally distrusted the process. This was in large part due to the side effects associated with receiving cowpox, despite their being far more benign than the effects of smallpox or previous methods of variola-tion.[15] Just as much of the population of Europe viewed with trepidation the notion of contracting one illness to prevent another, so too did the Filipinos in distant villages. While Balmis may not have witnessed the mass turn out of people that he experienced in Latin America, his efforts nevertheless led to the introduction of the vaccination process to Asia: "To deposit in these Islands that inexhaustible source of health, prosperity, and growth of population."[16] His humanitarian beliefs even took him to the Visayan archipelago, at that time in open revolt against the Spanish government.[17] Balmis continuously saw himself as having a mandate from humanity rather than simply from the crown.

Unfortunately, Balmis's combativeness combined with his own illness, as well as the governor-general's illness, hastened the end of the expedi-tion in the Philippines. With what he saw as little direct civil or religious support, the doctor who was mockingly referred to as Quixote by his adversaries in the Philippines decided to quit the islands.[18] The withdrawal largely involved only Balmis himself. Gutiérrez and others stayed behind to continue the process. Gutiérrez would remain on the islands for several years, eventually vaccinating some twenty thousand persons.

Balmis's decision to leave without the children he had brought from Mexico or his staff was driven by a number of factors. As the *Magallanes* was currently undergoing repairs, no suitable ship existed to ferry the expedition back across the Pacific. At the same time, the economic strain of the Napoleonic Wars had reduced the ability of the Philippine gov-ernment to continue funding the vaccination program.[19] Additionally, Balmis's deteriorating health and simultaneously deteriorating rela-tionship with Aguilar favored an early departure. The Spanish doctor undoubtedly saw his work in the archipelago as largely completed and hoped to take his efforts to the mainland and return to Spain to report on his achievements.

Fear of the side effects of the vaccination as well as of the dangers asso-ciated with travel to the Asian mainland unsurprisingly led to a lack of volunteers for the next leg of the voyage. While the arrival of the children from New Spain perhaps demonstrated the commitment of the Spanish to the health of their vaccine carriers, parents in the Philippines were less than eager to send their children to China. Balmis ultimately had to rely on the help of a priest from Santa Cruz who managed to find three boys for the weeklong trip to the Portuguese city of Macau on board the *Diligencia*. The shortest voyage of the expedition soon proved to be the deadliest. Beginning on the night of September 10 and continuing until September 15, a massive typhoon blanketed the South China Sea. The *Diligencia* was hit by strong winds and waves and nearly foundered on the rocks. Twenty lives were lost on the ship, as well as entire botanical collection belonging to the famed Scottish botanist William Kerr, who was then active in the region, before the ship finally arrived at the mouth of the Zhujiang River.

Balmis's initial target city was Macau. The Portuguese had received formal permission to settle the area in 1557 and quickly built a profitable trading port there. But as the seventeenth century progressed, conflicts with the Dutch and trade restrictions by the Qing and Tokugawa began a decline in Macau's importance and profitability. By the time of Balmis's arrival, the British were even considering seizing the location, allegedly to prevent French conquest but more generally because of its general neglect by Lisbon and Goa: "Macao is so little known . . . and . . . so neglected . . . that it is now the fit resort only of Vagabonds and Outcasts."[20] Despite this, the Spanish saw promise in maintaining good relations with the Portuguese and viewed the Iberian colony as a way to penetrate China.

The Portuguese leaders of Macau proved to be quite receptive to receiving the vaccination. Interest in Balmis's efforts were perhaps first kindled during his time in the Philippines and from the experience of various merchants who traveled between the two ports. One such example was Pedro Huet, commander of the Portuguese ship *Esperanza*, who had arranged for Balmis to vaccinate his crew. Upon the ship's arrival in Macau, these men disseminated information regarding the practice to both local authorities and the general population. The ship also attempted to introduce samples of the vaccine, but improper handling led to their destruction. Regardless, the attempt helped to create a local demand. In fact, the first two patients that Balmis treated upon landing were the city magistrate, Miguel José de Arriaga Brum da Silveira, and the archbishop-elect of Goa, Manuel de São Galdino. Governor Aguilar of the Philippines later nominated Arriaga to receive the Order of Charles III for his efforts to promote vaccination, a fitting award considering the monarch's support of exploration and the expansion of public health. Interestingly, a British doctor who belonged to the East India Company, George Staunton, had likewise brought the vaccine to China in 1805. The meeting of the two vaccines in the region demonstrated the rapidity with which scientific imperialism and European influence were circling the globe.

The final journey of the expedition saw the interaction of Balmis with the expanding British Empire. While still in Macau, he wished to bring the vaccination to China proper: "I had the pleasure of being the first to introduce the vaccine in the Chinese Empire." It remains telling of the state of the Middle Kingdom at the time that the country that originated the process of variolation almost a millennium before now saw the newest trend in public health arriving aboard a European ship. Unfortunately, leaders of the Royal Company of the Philippines, which controlled Spanish interests in the area, particularly Francisco Mayo and Martin Salaverria, proved less than enthusiastic about the undertaking. Because of this, the English at Canton took it on themselves to procure the vaccine, setting up a vaccine center in the city on December 2, 1805, and eventually transmitting the process to the court of the Jiaqing emperor, and "with this they opened a door to the heart of the Chinese."[21] This episode further demonstrated the ascendency of the British in Asia at the expense of the Spanish and Portuguese.

As for the children who crossed the Pacific, all twenty-five were returned to Mexico aboard the *Magallanes*. Their departure had been delayed by the repairs needed for the ship and a war scare in April of 1806, when the

British frigate *Greyhound* arrived off the coast of Manila. Finally arriving at Acapulco on April 19, 1807, the children were taken to the capital, and after meeting with the viceroy were eventually returned to their homes by the fall of that year. Rafael Gómez was placed in charge of this task and was responsible for supplying the children with food, clothing, and education as a royal reward for their actions. Only two boys of the original number were lost during the Pacific expedition, one in the Philippines and one after his return to Mexico City.

Following in the vein of previous Spanish expeditions, Balmis gathered hundreds of drawings and local plants from Asia for his return to Madrid. After building up a substantial collection, the Spanish doctor finally organized his return voyage. Boarding a Portuguese ship, the *Bon Jesus de Alem*, in Macau, he began the long journey back to the Iberian Peninsula. As the Spanish fleet had recently been destroyed by the British during the Battle of Trafalgar, his safety at sea could not be guaranteed. When the vessel needed to dock at the English-held island of Saint Helena, in the South Atlantic, Balmis selflessly readied vaccines for its citizens. Despite Spain and the United Kingdom formally being at war in 1806 as part of the War of the Third Coalition, the Spanish physician once again saw his mission as one of universal humanitarianism. Despite Balmis's eagerness, however, the governor of the island, Colonel Robert Patton, turned him down. Instead, Balmis left behind a package containing lymph material, instructions, and a handwritten letter to Edward Jenner that remained unopened for years.[22]

Undaunted, Balmis continued on his journey home, sailing north along the coast of Africa until he arrived in Lisbon in the summer of 1806. It had been nearly three years since he had left, having circumnavigated the globe and vaccinated hundreds of thousands of people on four continents. After requesting 750 pesos from the Spanish ambassador in the city, he hired a carriage and began the journey to the royal residence at Madrid. The doctor spent the rest of the year attempting to redress his financial expenses as well as have his plants and specimens from Asia brought in duty-free. When the latter was finally accomplished, he had the plants delivered to Francisco Antonio Zea, director of the Royal Botanic Gardens of Madrid. A story carried in the *Gazette* on October 14, 1806, summarized the extent of Balmis's expedition and offered a fitting eulogy to the undertaking.

On Sunday, September 7, recently past, Dr. Francisco Xavier de Balmis, honorary surgeon of His Royal Chamber, had the honor of kissing the hand of our King, having just traveled around the world with the sole purpose of bringing all the overseas domains of the Spanish Monarchy, and those of other diverse Nations, the inestimable gift of the Vaccine. His Most Serene Majesty, has been informed with the most intense interest of the main events of the expedition, showing himself extremely pleased that the results have exceeded the hopes that were conceived when undertaking it. This expedition, composed of several faculty members and assistants, and twenty-two children, who had not yet caught smallpox, destined to conserve the precious fluid, successfully transmit it from arm to arm from one to another over the course of the voyage, left the port of Coruna under the command of Balmis on Nov. 30, 1803. It first stopped at the Canaries, secondly at Puerto Rico, and thirdly at Caracas. After leaving this province for the port of Guayra it divided into two teams, with one set to travel throughout South America under the assistant director, Francisco Salvany; and the other under Balmis going to Havana, and from there to the Yucatan. In this province it again divided, with the professor Francisco Pastor heading to the port of Sisal to reach Villahermosa in the province of Tabasco and deliver the vaccine to Chiapas and Guatemala, heading down the long and rough road the 400 miles to Oaxaca, while the rest of the expedition, which arrived safely in Veracruz, not only traveled to the heart of the Viceroyalty of New Spain, but to the provinces beyond, from where it returned to Mexico City.[23]

The imagery of this Prometheus of vaccination and modern science kissing the hand of a king who represented a millennium-old monarchy that was close to crumbling before democratic revolution is a perfect portrayal of various elements of the expedition's place in history.

AFTERMATH OF THE EXPEDITION

Balmis's return to Spain and his efforts to capitalize on his expedition, both personally and in terms of pushing greater medical efforts and reforms, were complicated by the Napoleonic invasion. French forces had moved across the country in 1807 to prevent British machinations in Portugal. It was in this atmosphere that Balmis sought to continue his involvement in the politics of the nation. In February of 1807, he is mentioned as presenting a Spanish-Chinese dictionary to the secretary of state, Manuel de Godoy. A few months later, in June, we find Balmis petitioning for a position as chamber surgeon to Charles IV. Yet Franco-Spanish relations soon soured, and Balmis understandably largely disappears from Spanish events as the kingdom slowly collapsed into chaos around him.

Godoy's downfall in March of 1808 and the abdication of Charles IV led to increased French dominance in the capital. A subsequent citizen's revolt in May of 1808, though put down by force, soon led to the bloody and prolonged Peninsular War. Thousands were killed as the French engaged in violent repression against the towns of Spain in an attempt to end the guerrilla conflict. Balmis later reported that his own home had been sacked by the French. He had been "one of the first to follow the just cause of V. M., left his house and property, which were confiscated by the first decrees of the intruder King at his entry into this Capital."[24] Fleeing to Seville with other royalists, the Spanish physician split his time between engaging in efforts to support the king in exile and proposing new expeditions to vaccinate the colonies against smallpox. As part of the former, in August of 1808 he forwarded a copy of *Political Portrait of the Emperor of the French: His Conduct and that of His Generals in Spain, and the Loyalty and Courage of the Spaniards for Their Sovereign Fernando VII,* a book by Melchor Andario to his former companion Angel Crespo.[25] Because of this and other actions, it is not surprising to find Balmis's name on a list of persons whose property had been confiscated by the French in October of 1809.

Balmis had also heard around this time that, contrary to his explicit orders, the Mexican vaccination board had allowed the supply of vaccine material to fail. While he personally blamed this on the mismanagement of Viceroy Iturrigaray, the political situation and revolts in New Spain certainly played a role as well. In response, he petitioned the junta in Seville to commission a new expedition to the Americas. This was approved on November 30, 1809, and he immediately set about making arrangements for the voyage.

The ruling junta's reasoning in supporting Balmis is difficult to speculate. As the nation was in the middle of the Peninsular War, and the junta was fighting for its own survival and recognition, the decision to dispatch a medical expedition to New Spain seems a questionable use of time and treasure. Perhaps the answer lies in the current political situation in the Americas rather than in Spain. The abdication of Charles IV in March of 1808 and that of his son Ferdinand VII two months later created a legitimacy crisis in the colonies. Preexisting tensions between Criollos and Peninsulares were exacerbated and complicated by this power vacuum. Support among Spanish subjects in the colonies split among loyalty to Charles, Ferdinand, the ruling junta in Seville, and local authorities. The expedition could have been seen as a way to exert the junta's power in a way that was reminiscent of Charles's rule. The dispatch of medical care and scientific expeditions, after all, was a hallmark of Spanish Bourbon rule. Continuity of these efforts would help legitimize the junta.

The second Balmis Expedition left from Cádiz aboard the ship *San Fernando* in January of 1810. The boat departed in haste as a French army suddenly invaded Andalusia. The very junta that had approved the mission was soon dissolved, and Cádiz was placed under siege on February 5. On this trip, Balmis focused on a two-prong effort to restart the vaccination process in the Americas. First, he decided to bring a larger collection of Moreau's work on vaccination, arguing that it was the "lack of instruction" of the people that caused the inoculation efforts to grind to a halt after his and Gutiérrez's departure.[26] Second, to both reduce costs and depart more quickly, he chose to focus on finding samples of cowpox among the New World cattle and obtaining vaccine material from them. Numerous local governments and scientists had previously failed to discover the presence of the illness in Latin America. Part of Balmis's decision may have been influenced by the rapidly advancing French armies, which limited his ability to repeat the methods of his first expedition.

Balmis arrived at Veracruz several months later, and by May of 1810 was in Mexico City. During the summer of that year, he undertook efforts to examine the cattle of the Atlixco Valley, near Puebla, and modern-day Morelia, in Michoacán. By September he was back in Mexico City, unable to find infected cattle, and caught in the general uprising that followed the Grito de Dolores. Balmis instead focused his efforts on reforming the vaccine board that he originally created, drafting new proposals and regulations for its successful administration.

A second goal of the expedition was the fate of the orphans who had been transported to Mexico from Spain and the local children who had returned from the Philippine leg of the voyage. Contrary to the wishes of Charles IV and Balmis's own hopes, it appears that Viceroy Iturrigaray had failed to provide for their care and education. In June of 1810, Balmis addressed a letter to the Real Audiencia of Mexico City.

> I lived quietly in court, believing that what was sent was verified, when I received the complaints from the town halls and priests, as well as the representations of the parents and the children themselves . . . that nothing had been fulfilled of my promises, and that the viceroy, from the day after their arrival in Mexico, had returned them to their parents without giving them anything of what was promised. The intrusive French government was then in Madrid, and I had to suspend the impetus of my aching heart and wait for a

better chance to be able to represent the legitimate Spanish government, which was the Central Board that moved to Seville, where
I ran to look for it, taking with me the papers of the complaints
expressed.

Having heard all of the above, the junta deigned to send on behalf
of our sovereign Fernando Balmis to immediately remove from the
poor hospice the young children . . . and yet, that it has been more
than a year since it was issued, nothing has been accomplished, the
orphans still exist in the hospice, and those in the kingdom have
enjoyed nothing that has been sent by his serene majesty.[27]

Apart from the fate of the various children whom he had brought to
New Spain, as well as those whom he had transported across the Pacific,
Balmis also hoped to acquire news as to the fates of his former staff mem-
bers. Having left most of his assistants and doctors scattered across the
Americas, including Isabel Zendal, he began to press for information
regarding their whereabouts. Salvany's accomplishments and fate in South
America were also a mystery, with his death being unknown to Balmis
until March of 1813.

Zendal eventually received permission to settle with her son, Benito
Vélez, in Puebla, while Francisco and Antonio Pastor embarked for a
return to Spain in January of 1811. Attempts by Balmis to prosecute his
former associate Antonio Gutiérrez y Robredo for his apparent misspend-
ing of funds, failure to care for the orphans, and loss of two children on
the return trip to Mexico from the Philippines eventually came to naught
because of the political instability back in Spain. Gutiérrez remained in
New Spain and continued to practice medicine. Following the independence of Mexico, he was made a surgeon and professor at the national
university, showing the continued respect with which he was regarded by
the local community.

While opposed to the revolution taking place in Mexico, both for
political reasons and for its hindrances of his vaccination efforts, Balmis
also came into conflict with various conservative forces. In particular, a

feud developed between him and the bishop-elect of Michoacán, Manuel Abad y Queipo. Though the latter had been a staunch proponent of both variolation and vaccination, he quickly came into conflict with Balmis because of the Spanish doctor's approach to governance. A lawsuit even developed between the two men, largely based around Balmis's slandering of the bishop-elect.

By this point, the authorities in Mexico and Balmis himself were eager for him to return to Spain. Therefore, in August of 1811, his departure from New Spain was approved by the royal council. His first attempt to cross the Atlantic, on the ship *Ervinet*, failed because of the ongoing naval conflict in the oceans off the Americas. Finally, he was able to depart in late 1812 aboard the warship *Venganza*, docking in Cádiz in February of 1813.

His timing was fortuitous, as the year 1813 saw the return of the Spanish Bourbon monarchy to power and soon after the downfall of Napoleon. As an ardent supporter of the crown, a national hero, and a gifted self-promoter, Balmis spent the last several years of his life receiving accolades and awards. In 1814, he was appointed to the Royal Board of Surgery, and in June of 1815 was finally named a chamber surgeon, his lifelong ambition. He lived out the last several years of life in economic prosperity, dying on February 12, 1819, in Madrid at the age of sixty-five.

CHAPTER 10

The Impact of the Expedition

The light of the gospel and the Spanish name were spread everywhere.
—ANDRÉS BELLO, "ODA A LA VACUNA"

IT WAS NEVER BALMIS'S INTENTION or that of the Council of the Indies for the expedition to be an end in and of itself. The vast geography of the continents through which the expedition traveled, the cost involved, and the competing local interests would never have allowed for a full program of inoculation of the millions of Spanish subjects in the Americas and Asia. Rather, it was their hope that by beginning the process and by establishing vaccination boards, an apparatus could be put in place for eradicating smallpox over many years. Aside from the humanitarian aspect, improving the general health of the empire's population would deliver economic, military, and political benefits to the crown in the long run. While most investigations of the expedition end with its return to Spain, its impact on events abroad and on the practice of public health in subsequent years deserve a much more thorough investigation.

CONTINUING EFFORTS IN LATIN AMERICA

Experiences with improving public health in Latin America, specifically campaigns to inoculate the general public, varied greatly in the years immediately following the departure of Balmis and his fellow physicians from the region. While the majority of governors and viceroys continued to push for the practice, public opinion, financial constraints, institutional debates, and a looming revolution slowly enervated the movement.

Despite the tumult caused during Balmis's time in Puerto Rico, Governor Castro was eager to establish a permanent vaccine board upon the departure of the Spanish doctor and his staff. His efforts in seeking to acquire samples of the material even before the arrival of the Spanish expedition clearly demonstrate his interest in the process, one that continued following Balmis's removal. On August 22, 1804, shortly before he was replaced in power, Castro instructed the civic leaders of San Juan to undertake just such a program. Dr. Francisco Oller was tasked with discerning the logistical and medical requirements associated with the idea and quickly developed a plan that largely resembled those set up by the Spanish physician in Caracas and Mexico City. Vaccination houses were established, a proper census taken, practitioners trained, and reports of inoculations compiled. In keeping with José Flores's original design, local priests were instructed to encourage parents at their child's baptism to vaccinate them when they reached the proper age. Overall, Castro and Oller's efforts in Puerto Rico represent the epitome of the model designed by the Council of the Indies.

Vaccination appears to have continued in Puerto Rico over the next two decades, but in a sporadic fashion. The vaccine boards set up by Oller were less than persistent in their efforts, and new lymph had to be occasionally acquired from neighboring islands as the supply dwindled or was allowed to expire.[1] As the disease continued to erupt periodically, including in the capital city, it appears that many citizens were reluctant to undergo the process. In an effort to keep up with more modern notions of public health, new proposals were approved in 1818 by Governor Salvador Meléndez Bruna, and strict quarantine rules were placed on ships arriving with the illness. Even these moves proved to be less than totally successful, as new epidemics are recorded in 1855, 1863, 1871, 1873, 1875, and 1880. As late as the time of the American invasion in 1898, the *New York Times* explained that "the disease is endemic in Puerto Rico."[2] Finally, with the establishment of the Provincial Vaccine Institute in 1882, which increased the availability of preserved vaccine material, and an influx of money and medical support from America, smallpox was slowly eradicated on the island. The outbreak of several hundred cases in later 1898 and early 1899 prompted US military health officials to order the mass inoculation of Ponce.[3] At the same time, local efforts seem to have been succeeding, as a reporter for the *New York Times* reported in 1900 that, at least in San Juan, "freedom from sickness to a degree extraordinary in this latitude results . . . smallpox, and other tropical pests are virtually unknown here."[4]

The far wealthier and better organized island of Cuba tackled the illness with slightly more success. As previously mentioned, and continuing a pattern that dominated in the region, the island's governor, Salvador José de Muro, had been keen to eradicate the disease even before the arrival of Balmis. Shortly after Balmis's departure, a central vaccine board was set up under Dr. Tomás Romay y Chacón in 1804. A Criollo physician, Romay had spent years battling yellow fever on the island and eagerly took up the fight against smallpox as well.[5] Upon hearing of Jenner's discovery, he offered a prize of 400 pesos to whoever could bring the vaccine to Cuba or else discover cowpox among the island's cattle.[6] The arrival of María Bustamante and her household from Puerto Rico shortly before the arrival of Balmis in Havana seems to have been in response to this call.

The zeal Balmis demonstrated in spreading the process of vaccination in Cuba continued apace after his departure. By 1806, some 4,879 persons were vaccinated in Havana alone. A subsequent outbreak of the disease, spread by a recently arrived ship carrying enslaved people, quickly and predictably produced a panic among the citizens of the city. A young boy who jumped from the ship was taken to San Juan de Dios Hospital, only to succumb to smallpox shortly afterward. Fear of an epidemic pushed many to demand inoculation, and by the end of the year, some 16,000 were protected. Even after fear of contagion had dissipated, the procedure continued to be carried out by the central vaccination board. Between

1804 and 1835, it is estimated that some 311,342 people were inoculated on the island, representing perhaps 40 percent of the island's population at the time.[7]

Though the methods championed by Balmis and Romay continued to be practiced in Cuba for the next several decades, there were obvious limitations. Chief among these was maintaining an active supply of lymph material for use in the procedure. With the health of its enslaved labor being of the most importance to the ruling class in Cuba, the prevention and treatment of diseases like smallpox and yellow fever were given far greater consideration than in other parts of Latin America. In 1867, Dr. Vicente Ferrer traveled from the island to Europe to investigate recently developed methods of inoculation and vaccine preservation. Following his report, the royal government in Madrid approved payment on August 27, 1868, of the creation of the Practical Institute for Animal Vaccine of Cuba and Puerto Rico. Though aided by royal contributions, this was essentially a private scientific institution, the first of its kind in the Americas. Over the course of only a few years, the institute successfully inoculated twenty thousand individuals. As Ferrer was originally from Europe, he faced much of the same Criollo resistance and prejudice as Balmis did before him. Despite this, the vaccine campaign continued within the nation.

Unfortunately, a number of factors prevented the full eradication of the disease in Cuba. Chief among these were the superstitions of the population against the practice. Smallpox continued to be a significant scourge on the island for decades. By 1860, the government took even more drastic steps, mandating vaccination sweeps of infected neighborhoods in order to eliminate the pestilence finally and fully. By the time of the Cuban War of Independence, smallpox was still virulent and was cited as the second leading cause of death after yellow fever among Cuban and Spanish troops.[8] However, much of this was caused by the intermittent warfare of the latter half of the nineteenth century, and once independence had been achieved, the pestilence appears to have been under control. Though a journalist in May of 1899 praised the cleanliness of Havana and recounted that "there was not a case of smallpox or yellow fever in the city" as an attempt to promote American achievement since the occupation, it more likely revealed the accomplishments of almost a century of public health efforts by the Spanish and Cubans.[9]

As previously mentioned, while vaccination efforts in Mexico largely fell off after Balmis's departure, those in New Granada and Peru continued apace. After the departure of Balmis and Salvany from the region of Caracas, local physicians continued to provide inoculations. By November of 1805, Drs. José Domingo Díaz and Carlos del Pozo reported performing upward of thirty-seven thousand operations on local people. Del Pozo also wrote of discovering cowpox among the cattle of the region, allowing for a continuous supply of the vaccine and eliminating many of the problems experienced by vaccination boards in the Caribbean.

Díaz had an upbringing well couched in the ideas of the Enlightenment and the Scientific Revolution that characterized Balmis and others. Born in 1772 in Caracas, he studied medicine and surgery before graduating in 1795. During his time working at local hospitals in New Granada, he translated a copy of Benjamin Rush's work on yellow fever, hoping to incorporate many of its practices. Following the establishment of a central vaccination board in the city in 1804, Díaz was, not surprisingly, appointed as an early member. Working with Vicente Salias and del Pozo, he vaccinated tens of thousands before being forced to flee to Spain after Bolívar's revolution.

As was true in most other Latin American countries, the wars of liberation served to fragment and hinder the medical profession in New Granada. While men such as Antonio Vargas, educated in both Bogotá and Paris, attempted to piece back together the public health services of the newly independent South American states, vaccine programs fell by the wayside. In fact, medical knowledge in the region, affected by the nationalism of revolution, also became highly localized and distrustful of foreign ideas and methods.[10] This development would do much to undermine public health in Latin America.

Simón Bolívar, a victim of measles himself, was not opposed to improving public health. Smallpox occasionally ravaged his armies as they proceeded across the continent, a not uncommon occurrence but one he hoped to address. His letters, speeches, and dictates often spoke of the need of the new government to focus on the health needs of the people. During his final years as president of Gran Colombia, Bolívar decreed a law for the "Protection and Wise Use of the Nation's Forest Resources." The law presented as the impetus for its creation,

> First, that the Forests of Colombia, those owned publicly as well as privately, represent an enormous treasure in wood suitable for all types of construction as well as dyes, quinine, and other useful substances for medicine and the arts.
>
> Second, that throughout the region we are experiencing excessive harvesting of wood, dyes, quinine, and other substances, especially in the forests belonging to the state, with disastrous consequences.
>
> Third, that to avoid these, it is necessary to establish regulations for the effective protection of public and private property against violations of every kind, having seen the reports compiled for the government on this matter and heard the report of the Council of State.[11]

The subsequent decree called for cataloging all forests that contained useful medicine, especially quinine. After this, local juntas were to be set up to oversee the proper harvest and distribution of these to ensure their continual supply. These regulations extended to ports as well, injecting the government into the medical market. Interestingly, at least in the field of medicine, the new Spanish republic resorted to the restricted trade practices employed by the Habsburgs and Bourbons.

Farther to the south, an attempt by the newly independent nation of Chile to start its own vaccination campaign in 1830 failed miserably. Diego Portales, in his role as minister of the interior, had appointed

Doctor Guillermo Blest to develop a plan to vaccinate the nation. Portales went so far as to create a vaccination bureau in the style of Balmis and, when combined with the protocol developed by Blest, felt confident in his efforts to eradicate the disease.[12] But the assassination of Portales, the civil unrest and war that followed, and a lack of funding ultimately doomed the attempt. By 1881, the nation had only 350 doctors to care for a population exceeding two million.[13] Even when vaccines were offered, the response from the population often proved tepid at best. "Over half of the population, through ignorance or fear and prejudice, had refused to submit to the inoculation."[14] The effects of this became evident in 1871–72 when an outbreak of smallpox ravaged the country, killing in some parts upward of 41 percent of those infected.[15]

In the region of Peru, a similar story unfolded. Efforts by the royal governors to tackle issues of public health continued right up until the end of the revolution. In fact, Manuel Julián Grajales himself was captured by rebels while sailing up the coast of Chile aboard the *Thomas* in May of 1813. He had only recently been appointed head surgeon by the viceroy of Peru and was proceeding to the front. Thanks in part to his high standing in the region, however, Grajales was soon released.[16]

Much as it occured in Cuba and Puerto Rico, the new governor-general of the Philippines, Mariano Fernández de Folgueras, moved in 1806 to expand on Balmis's accomplishments. After helping to put down yet another local rebellion and further preparing the colony for possible involvement in the ongoing Napoleonic Wars, Folgueras established an insular bureau of vaccination that moved to spread inoculation to every island of the massive archipelago. By 1808, the local government was actively engaged on all major islands. The success of these efforts is demonstrated by the fact that in 1823, Dr. Fernando Casas claims that every town in the colony had seen the arrival of the vaccine.[17] Though the province did not experience the hindrances associated with rebellion experienced by the viceroyalties in the Americas, other internal and external forces hampered its efforts to spread the vaccine. Indigenous populations proved to be more resistant to actively participating in the practice. Overall, Folgueras's government was often required to resort to force and punishment to advance the process.

By the time of US annexation of the region, the disease was reported as prevalent in Manila and other cities. This could, once again, have been caused by over a decade of conflict and a breakdown in public health efforts. In fact, the islands saw the establishment of a vaccine production center in the 1850s and 1860s using local carabao calves, much as had occurred in Europe and Latin America. Likewise, detailed vaccine regulations were issued by the Spanish government there in 1851, 1873, and 1893. Regardless, local and US civil authorities moved quickly to reinstitute vaccination programs. By the middle of 1902, some three hundred thousand citizens in the region of the capital were reported as having undergone inoculation.[18] As with other American possessions, public health campaigns became a cornerstone of "benign assimilation."

The Spanish colonies were not the only ones to benefit from the actions of the Bourbons. Experiments with the practice of inoculation had continued in the Iberian Peninsula after the departure of the expedition. An article published in *El Reganon General* in February of 1804 not only demonstrated the reduced impact of smallpox during an outbreak that year but also assured its readers that "inoculation provides not the slightest harm to humanity."[19] In early 1805, as Balmis was arriving in the Philippines, the success of his enterprise in the Americas convinced Charles IV of the need to conduct a similar undertaking in Spain. As Felix Gonzalez wrote in 1814,

> Having thus the fullest knowledge of the subject at command, in all its breadth and extent, it [the committee] was able to lay before his Majesty the general results of vaccination, pointing out the probable means of giving perpetuity to this preservative until the much-to-be-desired extinction of smallpox in all regions and countries.[20]

The plan called for the establishment and maintenance of vaccine centers in all provinces, cities, and villages. An official proclamation, dated April 21, lays out the concerns of the king.

Our paternal affection towards our subjects being more than commonly excited by what has already been effected on arrival in the Canary Islands of an expedition intended by us to convey beyond the seas and propagate the discovery of vaccine, La Coruñah the admirable fruits thereof, in all our Indian dominions . . . I have now further resolved that there be in all Spanish hospitals . . . set apart and reserved in each a special ward for vaccination, to preserve and communicate vaccine to those who shall there present themselves . . . and that to the poor it shall be gratuitously given.[21]

The king's orders went on to lay out seventeen rules that would help to establish and preserve the practice in Spain. The following are the most important of the provisions:

RULE 1– Surgeons must perform gratuitous vaccinations on all who present themselves at a local hospital. This can be done only after establishing the fitness of the patient for the procedure.

RULE 2– All performances of vaccination must be registered and reported to the local government. These should then be compiled for the central vaccination board.

RULE 3– A standard model of a vaccination registry should be provided for all doctors to use.

RULE 4– All patients must be provided with a journal that they will use to track their health immediately following inoculation.

RULE 5– Surgeons must keep a journal of any anomalies that result from operations. These will then be presented every two months to their superiors to track any problems.

RULE 6– Senior surgeons will be tasked with training and advising junior staff.

RULE 8– Fathers of families will receive free vaccinations so as to financially benefit the family.

RULE 9 – Doctors and nurses must notify hospital administrators and the local junta of any problems that arise so the problems may be quickly and efficiently addressed.

RULE 10 – All hospital staff should be trained in the process so that they have a better understanding of it to communicate to the general population.

RULE 11 – All civilian leaders should actively promote the practice to the population.

RULE 12 – All ecclesiastical leaders should actively promote the practice to the population.

RULE 17 – The wealthy should be encouraged to donate money to local hospitals to cover the cost of vaccinating the poor.

Because of the necessities of war, the health of the Spanish army also received attention from both generals and the monarch. Toward the end of 1812, as the Peninsular War was at its height, Dr. Serapio Simces proposed that the soldiers of the Fourth Army be vaccinated against smallpox. The outbreak of a local epidemic among the soldiers in the region of Cádiz convinced the physician of the benefit of carrying out such a program. Intrigued by the suggestion, the government issued a royal order on January 3, 1813, recommending the voluntary mass vaccination of all soldiers in the nation.

THE WORLD'S RESPONSE TO JENNER AND BALMIS

Spain was not the only country to take an interest in the possibilities offered by Jenner's discovery. England had been at the forefront of the war against smallpox for a century. Beginning with Lady Montagu's discovery of variolation during her time in the Ottoman Empire in 1718, to Cotton Mather's writings and preaching in the English colonies, to Jenner's work eighty years later, the country and its citizens had been extremely active in seeking to eliminate the threat of this dreaded disease.

Like other parts of the globe, and despite being the birthplace of the smallpox vaccination procedure, the United Kingdom experienced much resistance to the practice among its citizenry. Regardless, the British government quickly grasped the economic and military application of vaccination. In 1802, it was made mandatory for all members of the British military to receive Jenner's treatment if they had not yet gotten smallpox. The disease had previously ravaged the English army during its time in the American Revolution, particularly during the Siege of Boston, and military planners hoped to avoid the same casualties during the Napoleonic Wars. This predated Spanish attempts by over a decade but followed a similar call by George Washington in the late 1770s. The American commander-in-chief wrote to William Shippen Jr., chief physician and director-general of the Medical Corps of the Continental Army, in 1777:

> Dear Sir: Finding the small pox to be spreading much and fearing that no precaution can prevent it from running thro' the whole of our Army, I have determined that the Troops shall be inoculated. This Expedient may be attended with some inconveniences and some disadvantages, but yet I trust, in its consequences will have the most happy effects.
>
> Necessity not only authorizes but seems to require the measure, for should the disorder infect the Army, in the natural way, and rage with its usual Virulence, we should have more to dread from it, than the Sword of the Enemy. Under these Circumstances, I have directed Doctr. Bond [Dr. Nathaniel Bond], to prepare immediately for inoculating this Quarter, keeping the matter as secret as possible, and request, that you will without delay inoculate all the Continental Troops that are in Philadelphia and those that shall come in, as fast as they arrive. You will spare no pains to carry them thro' the disorder with the utmost expedition, and to have them cleansed from the infection when recovered, that they may proceed to Camp, with as little injury as possible, to the Country thro' which they pass. If the business is immediately begun and favoured with

common success, I would fain hope they will soon be fit for duty, and that in a short space of time we shall have an Army not subject to this, the greatest of all calamities that can befall it, when taken in the natural way.[22]

By the middle of the century, amidst a flurry of other public health measures being passed at the time, the British Parliament officially began to move against the speckled monster. In 1840, the practice of variolation was made illegal, while vaccination was to be offered free of charge. This was followed up by the Vaccination Act of 1853, which mandated the practice for all children born in the country. Resistance continued in some quarters from ignorance, fear, or certain religious concerns. To combat this, subsequent vaccination acts were passed by Parliament in 1867, 1871, 1873, 1889, 1898, and 1907.

Other European countries followed in a predictable pattern. Bavaria mandated the practice for its citizens in 1807, and Denmark did the same three years later. The Central European states in general tended to have greater control over the public health of their citizens, and vaccination was practiced at a higher rate there than in England at the same time.[23] These efforts paid dividends during the Franco-German War, where only 457 out of 800,000 German troops died of the disease, while the French army saw 23,000 deaths, with many more in the general population.

Napoleon Bonaparte likewise approached the vaccine from a military perspective, realizing its potential to eliminate one of the frictions of war, as Carl von Clausewitz would later term them. Thus in 1804, we find the French emperor ordering the vaccination of his entire army. In fact, he personally called for a medal to be minted and presented to Jenner and even released several prisoners on Jenner's request. He would opine that he was unable to "refuse anything to one of the greatest benefactors of mankind."[24] Though Napoleon never made the process mandatory in France, he did publicly vaccinate his own son shortly after his birth, as an encouragement to the population. Thanks to his efforts, deaths in the nation from smallpox dropped from roughly 150,000 a year to around only 8,500. After

Napoleon's downfall, vaccination largely died off in the country with the restoration of the monarchy. Yet his efforts were not restricted to France only. At the same time the Spanish were pushing the practice in the New World, Napoleon was doing so among his conquered territories. This was particularly true in Italy, where over the course of a decade, close to one million inhabitants received the vaccine.[25]

In the United States, President Thomas Jefferson took an active interest in Jenner's discovery. Ever the scientist, Jefferson engaged Dr. Benjamin Waterhouse to test its efficacy. Waterhouse had first heard about the procedure in 1799 and acquired samples of the lymph a year later from an English practitioner. Immediately afterward, he vaccinated his wife and children. An exchange of letters and lymph material between the two men from 1800 to 1801 eventually convinced President Jefferson of the procedure's merits, and he soon after became a vocal proponent of it for the American population.[26] Writing to a relative of the English physician in 1806, Jefferson praised Jenner for his discovery and remarked on its importance.

> I have received a copy of the evidence at large respecting the discovery of the vaccine inoculation which you have been pleased to send me, and for which I return you my thanks. Having been among the early converts, in this part of the globe, to its efficiency, I took an early part in recommending it to my countrymen. I avail myself of this occasion of rendering you a portion of the tribute of gratitude due to you from the whole human family. Medicine has never before produced any single improvement of such utility. Harvey's discovery of the circulation of the blood was a beautiful addition to our knowledge of the animal economy, but on a review of the practice of medicine before and since that epoch, I do not see any great amelioration which has been derived from that discovery. You have erased from the calendar of human afflictions one of its greatest. Yours is the comfortable reflection that mankind can never forget that you have lived. Future nations will know by

history only that the loathsome small-pox has existed and by you has been extirpated.[27]

Despite Jefferson's support, vaccination tended to be a state issue within the country over the next century. Massachusetts became the first state to mandate the procedure for schoolchildren in 1855, with other states slowly following. By 1901, at the time of the famous *Jacobson v. Massachusetts* case regarding the constitutionality of mandatory vaccinations, the number of US states requiring vaccination had grown to only eleven. James Moore, writing on the history of vaccination in 1815, blamed the freedom of the nation and its citizens' belief in liberty for the slow and tortuous spread of inoculation there.[28]

Portugal had concerns similar to Spain's in terms of the political, social, and economic health of its American colony. Therefore, it is not surprising to find a similar undertaking of mass vaccination launched by Lisbon 1804. The physicians of the country seem to have become interested in Jenner's methods around the same time doctors in Spain had.[29] Yet it would take until March 1804 for the prince regent, Dom João, to agree to have his own sons vaccinated, thus starting the practice there. In the same year that Balmis crossed from Europe to the New World, a Portuguese ship was sailing in the opposite direction. Felisberto Caldeira Brant Pontes sent a vessel with enslaved children from Bahia to Lisbon in order to inoculate them. Pontes repeated Balmis's feat of bringing the children back across the Atlantic and using them to carry cowpox successfully to Brazil. By June 1, 1804, he reported having carried out the operation on 1,335 people in Bahia alone.[30]

China, though the birthplace of variolation centuries before, had experienced a collapse in the level of its medical advancement since the fall of the Ming dynasty. In a telling example of the rise of the West, it was European ships and doctors that helped to bring inoculation to the Qing Empire. Though the English East India Company (EIC) had privately attempted to bring the practice to Canton in 1803, the long sea voyage had rendered the sample useless. The arrival of Pedro Huet, along with his inoculated crew, as well as the visit of Balmis, helped to popularize the practice in Macao. Shortly afterward, Alexander Pearson, who served as a surgeon for the EIC, wrote a treatise on the practice that was subsequently translated into Chinese. Though Balmis and Pearson vaccinated only a handful of individuals in Canton, one of them, Qiu Xi, quickly began to practice the procedure himself.

Qiu Xi was born in 1774 in Nanhai County, outside of Canton. Though not a trained doctor, he took an interest in the medical arts and practiced locally in the Chinese community that coexisted with the Europeans in the great trading city. After being successfully vaccinated, he wrote a short work on the subject, *Yin dou lue* (Guiding the smallpox out), and then began to inoculate his family and others. Additional local physicians, including Liang Guochi, Zhang Yao, and Tan Guo, began to practice Jenner's method, a move financially supported by the local Hong merchants.[31] As in many of the Latin American nations, progress was slow and the inoculation material occasionally died out from lack of use, necessitating its import from British or Portuguese colonies in the region. Part of the reluctance arose from philosophical and scientific mistrust of the process and some from negative views of foreign technology. In order to help popularize the method, Qiu Xi published a collection of odes to the vaccine from survivors. Entitled *Yin dou ti yong*, it was compiled in 1823 and contained over 130 odes. Even the limited public embrace of a foreign technology was a milestone in the history of Chinese science and its view of its place in the world.[32]

From Eurasia to the Americas, the vaccination of the public against smallpox was handled quite differently based on several factors. While some nations seized the process early on, others left it up to the people to secure their own health against the disease. At the same time, opposition to vaccination, based on numerous factors, arose around the globe, and cannot be attributed to one simple cause. Some religious groups pushed back against the process, and others fully embraced it. Likewise, scientists and the general public both were split on the merits of vaccination. Regardless, the process slowly worked, and by the twentieth century, smallpox was rapidly on its way out in the developed world.

Interestingly, Spain itself experienced a falling off of the practice of inoculation. The political collapse of the nation into several decades of revolution and instability saw a similar decline in the quality of public health in the country. In fact, by 1814, because of the strain of the Peninsular War, "Spain, carefully planted with local vaccine institutions, indoctrinated with ideas of this hygienic propaganda, had become so dull in all her instincts as to the preservation of human life that she became dependent on a single individual, and he of little note, for the continuance of vaccination in her territory."[33] The fact that the physician Gil y Albenoz is said to have possessed the only source of lymph material in the peninsula at this time, only a decade after the Balmis Expedition's initial departure, clearly shows the nadir that public health efforts in Spain had reached. Even the government's revolutionary decision to order the mass vaccination of the army as an impetus to total public vaccination soon fell by the wayside, as similar orders had to be issued in 1832, 1848, and 1851.[34] Finally, Charles IV's own nephew, Infante Don Pedro Carlos, died of the disease in 1812 while in exile in Brazil, a fate similar to what had befallen both his parents in 1788.

The surest proof of this failure to continue Charles IV's vision was the outbreak of a major smallpox epidemic in the nation in 1866. Coming in the waning days of the reign of Isabella II, the pestilence eventually spread to all major cities of the Iberian Peninsula. Foreign observers were quick to point toward the recent decline in Spanish medical interventionism, "a censurable abandonment of vaccine lies clearly at the root of the disaster."[35] Though medical officials in Madrid, most notably Francisco Miguel Cuadrado, worked tirelessly to end the outbreak, the Spanish population had become largely hesitant of vaccination, a complete volte-face from the start of the century.[36] This outbreak was followed by a more general European one from 1870 to 1874, spread in part by the Franco-German War.

This decline in the vaccine's use can also be attributed to several additional factors. Most notable among these was the concurrent rise in syphilis rates. Arm-to-arm transmission of smallpox lymph served as vector of this reemerging illness. The occurrence of several notable episodes during the American Civil War, as well as in southern Italy, did much to drive people away from vaccinations by the middle of the century.[37] The rise and acceptance of the germ theory of transmission likewise helped to doom Jenner's process of vaccination as physicians sought more hygienic methods by which to inoculate patients.

SCIENTIFIC ABSOLUTISM AND LATIN AMERICAN REVOLUTIONS

Despite the humanitarian nature of the expeditions of both Charles III and Charles IV, the rise of scientific absolutism exacerbated the growing divisions between Spain and its colonies. As previously mentioned, the various scientific missions that traversed Latin America during the eighteenth century did much to extend Europe's knowledge of the plants and animals of the region. Likewise, the Europeans' use of the latest Linnaean system of classification helped to establish connections between the flora and fauna of both hemispheres. Yet the efforts drew criticism from local residents and scientists.

The acceptance of a general scheme of classification meant the replacement of traditional, varied, and local schema. For the Indigenous and Mestizo population of the Spanish colonies, this could be viewed as another example of imperialism, of forced cultural assimilation. More traditional Native names for plants and animals were being replaced by Latin names, much as the Church had replaced local deities and practices. Scientific uniformity was creating cultural uniformity.

At the same time, conflict arose even between the educated physicians of the New World and those of the Old. The methods and beliefs of Balmis, Salvany, and others may have differed only slightly from those practiced by Oller and Juan Marimón, but the attitudes of the former, particularly of Balmis, produced resentment among the latter. The vast majority of medical practitioners in New Spain, New Granada, and Peru were Criollos, with most being educated at universities in the colonies. These universities and their degrees were viewed with condescension by those trained in Iberia. The tension that already existed between the elite in the various viceroyalties and those in Spain now spread to the medical community as well.

A telling example of this involved the aforementioned Dr. Vicente Ferrer. Though his research and discoveries helped to advance inoculation methods in Cuba during the 1860s, his status as a Peninsular led to conflicts with local physicians.[38] As Dr. S. H. Gonzalez points out in her study of the changing nature of vaccination programs in late nineteenth-century Cuba, local resistance to Ferrer's then-radical views coalesced into a form of nationalism. Pride in the Criollo-dominated vaccine board was mythologized and glorified and used to push revolutionary agendas against control by Madrid.

Similar examples abound throughout Latin America, as can be seen in Balmis's interactions with various doctors and civil leaders. Even in Mexico City, where the vaccine was acquired largely through the work of the Peninsulares Iturrigaray and Arboleya, the implication that the various regions of the Western Hemisphere could acquire lymph material and manage their own inoculation programs without Madrid became a rallying cry for local revolutionaries in the lead up to independence from Spain.

Salvany, though much less hostile in his direct dealings with local physicians and civic authorities than Balmis was, was still viewed with harsh suspicion. One historian notes that "many doctors viewed Salvany as an outsider who knew nothing about Peru and the country's diseases, and they were quick to dismiss his ideas."[39] This local opposition, which hinged more on Criollo nationalism and thoughts of inferiority than on actual medical concern, was merely a scientific version of the larger revolutionary political debates then taking place.[40] Men like José Ignacio Bartolache tended to be from less well-off families "and rose to higher levels in society thanks to education."[41] As such, they tended to view the elite doctors of Europe as a threat to their legitimacy and were in turn discounted by them. Especially in Peru, where local attempts to acquire the vaccine had predated Salvany's arrival, "doctors had declared the vaccine a creole medical triumph."[42] A similar division took place in US medicine during the yellow fever epidemic of 1793, where the views on disease and treatments by such medical practitioners as Benjamin Rush and Adam Kuhn split as much along socioeconomic and political lines as by actual scientific debate.

In fact, many of the physicians and leaders whom Balmis and Salvany encountered in their journeys would eventually become notable revolutionaries. Included among these was Vicente Salias, who worked with Dr. Díaz in New Granada after Balmis's departure. Apart from founding the Sociedad Patriótica de Caracas, Salias allegedly also penned the first verse of what would become the Venezuelan national anthem. After fighting by the side of Simón Bolívar for a number of years, Salias was eventually executed in 1814. Thus, these men's preexisting political hostility toward Spain became entwined with their scientific and medical opposition as well.

Many in the Church who were encountered by the expedition were likewise split in their support for the future of Latin America. Juan Marimón, the priest and doctor who so actively welcomed and encouraged Balmis during his time in Cartagena, moved to support the uprisings in the region. In a similar vein, Andrés María Rosillo y Meruelo, the priest in Bogotá who praised Salvany's arrival, would also go on to side with the Criollo revolution.

In fact, of those doctors and civic officials who came into contact with the expedition, only José Domingo Díaz emerged as a staunch supporter of the royalist movement during the wars of independence. Though an orphan who was raised and educated in Caracas and a partner of Salias in his vaccination program, Díaz chose to side with the king against the independence of New Granada. This can perhaps be explained in part by the fact that he traveled to Spain to finish his education and received an official appointment a few years after Balmis's departure, making him more tied to the peninsula for his success. Upon Díaz's return to New Granada in

1810, the new revolutionary junta refused to recognize his credentials. Díaz fought for the royalist cause before being forced to flee to Puerto Rico in 1821.

Overall, the Balmis Expedition both increased preexisting rifts between Spain and its colonies and created new ones in the medical and scientific fields. Its success helped to inspire similar progress in Latin American medicine as well as in the medicine of other nations. Yet the scientific absolutism that accompanied the expedition did much to undermine these efforts over the next several decades. Millions of lives were likely saved, and many more were driven toward freedom and independence by the means of cowpox.

CHAPTER 11

Damnatio Memoriae

Look on my Works, ye Mighty, and despair!
—PERCY BYSSHE SHELLEY

ANDRÉS BELLO, THE GREAT SOUTH AMERICAN HUMANIST, amongst his myriad political and personal writings, composed a lengthy ode to the vaccine expedition that traversed his homeland. Among the many celebratory lines in the work, he exclaims that "the light of the gospel and the Spanish name were spread everywhere." To Bello, the expedition was not simply a scientific undertaking but a humanitarian one grounded in the truest notions of Christianity. It was an expedition that brought credit to Spain and its monarchy as well as to the Christian faith. Though perhaps an odd choice of topic for a poem, the magnitude of the undertaking and its humanitarian undertones appealed to a man whose life straddled the Enlightenment and the Romantic era. Bello had actually served as a secretary for the vaccine board of New Granada starting in 1807 and began his political aspirations in this position before going on to tutor the young Simón Bolívar.[1] His early experience with the crown in New Granada was generally favorable and certainly left him in awe of the power of both the king and science.[2] His poem was as much a paean to Charles IV and Balmis as it was to the accomplishments of man.

After describing the nearly apocalyptic destruction caused by the outbreak of smallpox in the region and praising Jenner for developing a cure, Bello goes into a lengthy ode to the glory of Charles IV.

Carlos sends; at this point a glorious
expedition which diffuses in his vast
domains the immense benefit
of that great and happy discovery.
He uses treasures from his treasury;
and stimulated with the high example
of royal piety,
all patriotic bodies are invigorated with zeal.
He chooses enlightened teachers
and a wise director, who, to his performance
of such an honorable office, contributes
his cares, lights, and talent.
Illustrious expedition! The most illustrious
to the amazement of the times
it will forever be recognized by humanity;
and whose salutary effects,
in the most remote age hence,
will be measured with the same level of amazement,
the sands from the Ponto,
or the stars which number from the sky.

Though Balmis is mentioned by name only once in the poem, the clear respect and appreciation paid by the author to both the doctor and the king of Spain are unique at a time of political insurrection against the rule of Spain. Perhaps Bello could defend his admiration in terms of his subjects representing the pre-Napoleonic regimes of Spain rather than the current rulers who were being risen against. The ideals of the vaccine expedition, of a caring government using the most modern science to benefit the common man, were worthy of song and poem. Likewise, Bello may have hoped that this model could serve as an inspiration to the current and future leaders of New Granada.

Several thousand miles away, in England, Edward Jenner spoke and wrote several times on the expedition. The English physician appreciated the humanitarian nature of the undertaking, famously opining, "I don't imagine the annals of history furnish an example of philanthropy so noble, so extensive as this." Despite his country being locked in war at the time with France and Spain, Jenner accepted the praise heaped on to him by Napoleon and Balmis for his part in helping to eradicate the disease. He later recounted to a friend, "I have made peace with Spain and quite adore her philanthropic monarch."[3] In the same vein, the great explorer Alexander von Humboldt wrote, "This expedition will permanently remain as the most memorable in the annals of history."[4]

For Spain and her imperial possessions, the expedition had been a profound success. It is estimated that by 1815, 10 percent of the Spanish population in Iberia alone, some one million souls, had been vaccinated against smallpox.[5] Perhaps an equal number had been saved from the disease in the Americas and Asia. The potential loss of taxation, labor, and offspring from smallpox deaths would have been enormous. Spain was once again at the forefront of medical science and had revolutionized and expanded the focus of public health efforts on the global stage. Undoubtedly, a large percentage of the population of Latin America and the Philippines today is descended from those who were saved by Charles IV and Balmis.

Apart from speeches and poems, several monuments were erected at the time to Spain's accomplishments. In the Philippines, these included a historical marker at the Research Institute for Tropical Medicine at Alabang, and a statue of Charles IV in the Plaza de Armas in Manila, across from the Metropolitan Cathedral of the Immaculate Conception. The statue was commissioned and installed in 1824 and complemented with a fountain in 1886. In the Canary Islands, a statue of Father Manuel Díaz was put up outside the Church of El Salvador, in the Plaza de España, to commemorate his efforts in supporting the vaccine program as well as his general accomplishments while on the island. Even in Mexico City, the former provincial capital whose leaders had given Balmis considerable resistance, a street was named for Balmis in the newly laid out Colonia

Doctores section in the late nineteenth century. Interestingly, the Hospital General de México was founded on the street in 1905, a very fitting location for such an institution.

Yet very quickly the expedition seems to have disappeared from the collective memory of much of the planet. Even in Spain itself, Balmis and his mission were either forgotten or employed as a watchword for the misapplication of resources by the Bourbon government. Concerning public health, Felix Gonzalez, a contemporary writer, asked, "What have we done for the present generation in this thing of first importance? Nothing."[6] By the middle of the century, the prevailing opinion in England was of a Spain that was totally ignorant of vaccination and modern medical science. A journal at the time carried the generally accepted view of a "Spain, which is so much behind the rest of Europe in all mental acquirements."[7] American histories of the era, such as Hubert Bancroft's *History of Mexico* (1852) and Frederick Ober's *Popular History of Mexico* (1894), lack any mention of the expedition, with the latter referring to Charles IV as "weak and dissolute" and "corrupt . . . despicable."[8] Various Mexican books on the history of the region, including Lucas Alamán's multivolume *Historia de Mexico* (1840s), Tirso Rafael Córdoba's *Historia Elemental de Mexico* (1881), and Francisco Banegas Galván's *Historia de Mexico* (1923), either fail to include even a brief footnote to the expedition or mention it merely in passing.[9]

Even in the Philippines, the reason behind the casting of a statue of Charles IV and its placement in the Plaza de Armas, now the Plaza de Roma, was soon forgotten. Following that nation's independence, the monument was even removed during the nationalistic years of the 1960s and replaced with one depicting the three Filipino priests, Mariano Gómez, José Burgos, and Jacinto Zamora, collectively known as Gomburza, who had been executed by the Spanish in 1872 following the Cavite Mutiny. It would take until 1981 for the statue of the Spanish king to be returned to its original place of installation.

How was the expedition termed by Jenner as "an example of philanthropy so noble, so extensive" so quickly stricken from the collective memory of most of the planet? Why especially was this the case in Latin America and Spain, locations where it would be expected to be particularly remembered and celebrated? Why was it not more widely celebrated in the medical community? The answers perhaps lie in the series of events that immediately followed the expedition.

Beginning with a collection of minor rebellions and the establishment of juntas in 1808 and 1809, wars of independence erupted across Latin America that did not end until the formal independence of Bolivia in 1825. For a number of reasons, these conflicts did much to help erase Charles IV and Balmis's story from the historical record in the region. As has been previously shown, the vaccine effort met with resistance from local Criollos, which helped to exacerbate growing splits between the colonies and Spain. For the local elite in the New World, Balmis's scientific absolutism and previous expeditions were further proof of Madrid's domineering power. The examples of Dr. Francisco Oller y Ferrer in Puerto Rico, Alejandro Arboleya in Mexico, and Pedro Belomo in Peru could all be used by nationalists to show that inoculation would have emerged without the direct intervention of Spain. Oller's efforts in particular stand out as his approach embraced the concept of free trade and helped bring the vaccine across the Caribbean and to New Spain. Therefore, local physicians could pride themselves on having solved the problem, making Balmis, his efforts, and Bourbon interventionism largely unnecessary. Others chose to follow a different path of revisionism, arguing that it was their local Criollo efforts that inspired Balmis and Charles IV in the first place.[10] The subsequent expulsion of Peninsulares from many of the newly formed countries likewise played into this shift toward denigrating the contributions of Spaniards and praising those of local agents.

At the same time, for almost all classes in Latin America, it was necessary to portray Bourbon rulers as incompetent or tyrannical. Revolutionary propaganda demanded that the monarch be blamed for the problems in the colonies, problems that could be solved only through local, democratic action. Thus we find the Grito de Dolores's push for an end to bad government, its denunciation of Spain, and its call for "death to the gachupins." Spain, its kings, and its viceroys were the authors of all evils, not benefactors of the people. Acknowledgement of Spanish beneficence would have cut against this narrative. This is comparable to efforts by many in the newly formed republic of the United States to distance themselves from England and its contributions.

Finally, the Spanish king's philanthropy presented an economic issue for many within the colonies. As was previously mentioned, many local physicians and inoculators resented Balmis and Salvany because of the financial impact the Spanish doctors would have on their businesses. The well-meaning efforts of Charles IV and his royal surgeons were at odds with the marketplace in medical care in the region. Though the Bourbon reforms had pushed for expanded internal free trade within the empire, they still fell far short of the rights accorded to British colonial merchants and well below the total free trade demanded by revolutionaries in America. Balmis's disruption of the medical market would have added to the anti-Spanish sentiment already brewing in the region.

Following independence, these beliefs continued and were subsumed by a nationalist rewriting of history. Part of this took place in the form of efforts by Latin American nations and individuals within them to claim credit for the success against smallpox in the first decade of the nineteenth century and for the launching of the expedition in the first place. This was most readily seen in Salvany's interactions with the various Criollo doctors of Lima. One notable resident, the wealthy merchant Matías Larreta, stated at the time that he had personally developed a plan to transport the vaccine across the ocean using orphans, months before Flores and Balmis had: "In response to the request made in my name for these purposes, [Charles IV] expressed his sovereign will to make this inestimable project a royal one."[11] Larreta had previously been involved with the Malaspina Expedition, helping to transport its discoveries back to Spain.[12] Conversely, most of the nations of Latin America saw an immediate, rapid decline in public health efforts that had been established under Spanish rule. With the slow recovery of these institutions over the next few decades by *higienistas*, a sense of nationalistic pride in health care emerged.[13] The various democratic leaders and caudillos of the region were likewise quick to seize on any medical developments as propaganda for their administrations. History necessarily had to be rewritten, then, to portray the seventeenth and eighteenth centuries as a medical dark age, with the actions of these new governments in the nineteenth century serving to improve the human condition. Finally, the failure of many of the post-independence regimes to solve the region's inherent socioeconomic problems necessitated a rewriting of history in an attempt to blame conditions on the pre-revolutionary actions of Madrid and local governors. The new presidents and caudillos, therefore, had merely inherited nations in untenable conditions.

This academic development fit in well with the concept of the Black Legend. Centuries of English and Protestant propaganda had portrayed the Spanish as brutal conquerors who brought nothing to the New World except death and slavery. Even after the extent of smallpox as a decimator of Indigenous populations rather than Spanish swords became well established, Madrid was still held liable by many for the disease's arrival and spread in the New World. As a later history falsely claimed, "Though the Spaniards themselves do not appear to have suffered much from this dread disease they were the means of bringing it to this unhappy country."[14] The view of Spain as an unholy empire was soon joined by a view of it as a backward and primitive region. Examples of this attempted revisionism became more prominent as the expedition once again became more well known. A news article published in 2014 chose to focus on the role of the queen and Manuel de Godoy as the main force pushing for the launch of the mission, referring to Charles as "a masterpiece of kingly mediocrity: stout and bovine, well-meaning but lacking nerve, indifferent to the affairs of the state but fiercely loyal to the institution he represented, solemn and simple-minded, a prodigious begetter of heirs and a perfectly ineffectual sovereign."[15] This was a view proposed by many modern Spanish historians in the twenty-first century.[16] Holding this view of Charles would then necessitate either a denigration of the Balmis Expedition or a move to attribute it to someone else.

Likewise, the historical efforts of the Catholic Church in combating disease were glossed over by Protestant writers and theologians. Works produced for English-speaking and Protestant audiences tended to focus on the brutality of the Spanish reign in the Americas. Frederick Ober succinctly encapsulated the Anglo-American view of Spanish rule over the Americas as "three centuries of oppression."[17] Taken to the other extreme, the Catholic Church's embrace of inoculation ran afoul of many Protestant groups that opposed the practice for religious reasons. As seen by the levels of violence experienced by Cotton Mather in Boston, the act of vaccination itself was a source of contention that was used to tarnish the image of those who practiced it. For two centuries, British and American historians chose to portray Spain during the fifteenth to eighteenth centuries as either a cultural and intellectual backwater or as a destructive empire.

The rise of ideologically far left political parties and interest groups in the twentieth and twenty-first centuries has expanded the Black Legend to be a denunciation of most Western, capitalist, and premodern efforts. In this historiographical environment, the philanthropy of the Balmis Expedition and the various scientific and beneficial endeavors of Charles III and Charles IV do not fit the general narrative. Even when they are present, they tend to be portrayed in a negative light as examples of imperialism, as merely for economic gain, or as a paltry attempt to combat a problem created by the Spanish in the first place. In March of 2019, Andrés Manuel López Obrador, the new president of Mexico, began his term by seeking an apology from the current king of Spain, "to ask forgiveness of Indigenous peoples for violations of what are now known as human rights."[18]

A nineteenth-century English journal nicely sums up this attitude: "However much our pride may feel a hurt that a power, even then on the decline, whose maritime influence and wealth has paled before that of

Britain, should have taken so leading a part in bringing into use and operation this product of an English soil."[19] Rising nationalism and a hatred for everything Spanish, especially in England and the Americas, made it taboo to praise or even mention the efforts of Francisco Balmis. In fact, many English writers and physicians even began to publicly question the success of the Spanish in the endeavor, proclaiming Balmis and his men to be "quacks."[20] Once again, the ability of those in the New World to undertake vaccinations themselves was emphasized, or the event was seen as a limited function with no impact on the future of the various nations.

Part of this arose from a desire on the part of Anglo-Saxon nationalists in the nineteenth century to praise Jenner's accomplishments. His discovery was given a mythological status and all subsequent vaccination efforts, whether foreign or domestic, were seen as merely outgrowths of his initial achievement. Thus emerged an almost gnostic, Mandaean shift, pushing John the Baptist to the front of the faith. Lord Byron himself, while writing his epic poem that took place in Spain only a decade after the launching of the expedition, makes no mention of efforts by Madrid to counter the disease but does lavish praise on Jenner.

> What opposite discoveries we have seen!
> (Signs of true genius, and of empty pockets.)
> One makes new noses, one a guillotine,
> One breaks your bones, one sets them in their sockets;
> But vaccination certainly has been
> A kind antithesis to Congreve's rockets,
> With which the Doctor paid off an old pox,
> By borrowing a new one from an ox . . .
> I said the small-pox has gone out of late;
> Perhaps it may be follow'd by the great.[21]

As previously mentioned, almost no scholarly materials on either side of the Atlantic included the expedition in their general histories of the region or in histories of medical evolution. The first major work for even a Spanish audience on the topic of the expedition, Gonzalo Díaz de Yraola's *La vuelta al mundo de la expedición de la vacuna*, would not be published until 1948. Even in academic journals, save for several articles by Professor S. F. Cook in the 1940s, Balmis remained a relatively obscure topic until the turn of the twenty-first century.[22]

Balmis himself presaged his fate, and that of his expedition: "They call it glory, to devastate everything and make men suffer . . . monuments are raised to these villainous triumphs, and on them people lavish their applause."[23] But beginning around the turn of the twenty-first century, interest once again arose around Balmis and the vaccine expedition. In fact, several historical novels on the subject have been published in recent years, including *A flor de piel* by Javier Moro, which sold over two million copies worldwide. In time for the two-hundred-year anniversary of its launch, the expedition was finally honored with a monument in the city of La Coruña. Interestingly, while Balmis and the facts of his voyage are included in the open-air exhibit at the Museo Domus, the majority of the site is dedicated to the orphans who accompanied him, as well as to their nurse, Isabel Zendal. A focus on popular history and a movement away from the historiography of "the great man" can be seen in these decisions.

Because of the needs of the revolutionaries in Latin America, the political goals of the caudillos and leaders that followed the independence movement, the continuance of the Black Legend by Anglo-American historians, and the push to Marxism in the region during the twentieth century, Spain's great accomplishments, particularly those of the Balmis Expedition, fell by the wayside. As is often stated, history is written by the winners, and with the downfall of the Bourbons, their supporters found that their achievements had become inconvenient in the newly accepted chronology of events.

Yet, as John Adams once opined, "facts are stubborn things." In the end, whether wittingly or not, the Balmis Expedition inspired a series of similar efforts aimed at eradicating disease on the planet, and, slowly, more information on the original model for those undertakings has come to the attention of the public. By the early twentieth century, most developed nations were actively vaccinating their populations against myriad threats to humanity. By the start of the Cold War, most worldwide efforts focused on the elimination of disease moved toward Latin America, Africa, and parts of Asia. Interwoven with notions of humanitarianism, economic concern, political necessity, and Cold War politics, these efforts closely paralleled those of Charles IV. Campaigns by the United Nations and George W. Bush's PEPFAR initiative can all be viewed as twentieth- and twenty-first-century versions of Balmis's Expedition. Many of these campaigns proved just as controversial as their original model had been, yet their long-term impact on the future of humanity is unquestionable. The efforts of Charles IV, Balmis, and dozens of orphans helped to save untold millions of lives and stand as a triumph to Spain, the medical arts, and humanity.

Conclusion

DISEASE HAS BEEN PERHAPS the greatest change agent in human history. Illness has affected the development of civilization, guided the destiny of kingdoms, and led to the deaths of billions of humans. For thousands of years, it has served as both a limiting agent and a catalyst for growth. The Neolithic Revolution produced an explosion in human population and led to the concentration of people in permanent settlements. While bacteria, parasites, and viruses have always plagued the human species, the consequences of this stage in human development helped to exponentially increase the problems of disease. Civilization, in many ways, produced disease. As humanity expanded around the globe, increasing the size of empires, opening trade routes, and increasing interactions among different societies, disease became pandemic. The modern era has not ended the problem. While many diseases have been eradicated or have become treatable, and while diseases of affluence have largely replaced the more primitive ones, disease remains an ever-present killer. Over the 2017/18 flu season alone, some seventy-nine thousand Americans died of the disease, nearly five times the number of people killed by guns that same year, twice the number killed by cars, and nearly equal to the number that died of poisonings.[1] Likewise, the more recent pandemic that started in 2019, COVID-19, has shown that the world is not yet removed from the ravages of a massive worldwide plague.

At the same time, the onslaught of disease helped to push human development further along, serving as a catalyzing agent to modernization. The presence of illness led to developments in religion, sanitation, art, technology, science, and, most notably, medicine. While Heraclitus's dictum that war is the father of all may be accurate, disease should then be considered the creative mother figure. Its horrors inspired creation out of brutal necessity.

Spanish history, like that of any other nation, is awash with pestilence. The diseases that helped to topple the Roman Empire had an equal impact on the population of the Iberian Peninsula, paving the way for Visigothic occupation and later Islamic conquest. Disease also touched on many important moments in the history of the medieval Spanish monarchy. At the same time, the presence of illness pushed both the Catholic Church and local Islamic organizations to fund the creation of hospitals to care for the population. The fact that both traditions existed in geographic proximity to each other allowed for an exchange of ideas and competition in practices as well. As seen in the example of Alfonso X, a more practical and scientific approach to medicine dominated much of the history of the peninsula.

The Habsburg and Bourbon dynasties were as affected by disease as any other family living in Europe at the time. In the case of the former, generations of close marriages severely weakened the genetic diversity of the ruling family and led to a number of chronic and inherited physical and mental deficiencies. Ultimately, disease brought down the Habsburg dynasty and allowed for the ascension of the Bourbons. This new dynasty proved to be no more immune to the ravages of disease than their cousins had been. The various Spanish monarchs of the eighteenth century lost the majority of their children, including heirs to the throne, to illness. The royal family of Spain was as affected by disease and as concerned with the issues of public health as the general population was.

The handling of public health issues in Spain did not begin with the advent of the Enlightenment and the rise of absolutism, but it had its roots in the actions of both the Catholic Church and the Caliphate of Córdoba. The construction of charity hospitals and efforts to treat the ills of the public were already ongoing as the Renaissance dawned in the region. The subsequent influx of Enlightenment notions of the role of government in treating illness and the advent of the Scientific Revolution merely magnified preexisting trends in Spain.

Spain's history and geography made it central in the flow of diseases into and out of Europe. Endemic smallpox and typhus appear to have first entered the continent through the Iberian Peninsula, largely because of the region's involvement with wars in the Near East. Likewise, Spanish exploration of the New World spread diseases that ultimately killed over 90 percent of the Indigenous population there. These returning conquistadores then possibly brought syphilis to Spain and Italy, resulting in a pandemic that soon reached even Japan. The diseases inadvertently spread by the development and growth of Spain resulted in the deaths of hundreds of millions of people and dramatically shaped the political, economic, social, and religious future of the world.

While the Spanish Empire, like all others in history, existed to empower and enrich itself, several factors led it to become a far more benign imperial power than it is often portrayed to be. The Reconquista was pursued not only through military means but also through the conversion and inclusion of local conquered populations. Demographic necessity then saw this process repeated in the New World after the arrival of Columbus. With disease decimating the local population and migration from Iberia being far below the levels that would be seen following the arrival of the English a century later, Spanish rulers attempted several methods by which to employ, convert, and adopt the local Indigenous people.

From the earliest attempts at settlement, the Spanish sought to transform the new lands of the Americas into Spain. Universities and hospitals, the highest signs of civilization at the time, were constructed within the first few decades of Spain's arrival. By comparison, with the exception of Harvard, colleges were not established by the English colonists until nearly the eighteenth century, and the first major public hospital would not be built there until 1751. Though the strict caste system established by the Spanish has been repeatedly criticized, it did at least allow for the intermixing of races and provided a place and role for all people in the society. Between the active presence of the Catholic Church and the Spanish attempts to incorporate the local population, the health and well-being of the inhabitants became an early concern.

Nor did the Spanish monarchs benignly neglect their colonies. Instead, they took an active role in developing and exploring them. Charles III launched numerous expeditions in the eighteenth century. Influenced by absolutism and notions from the Enlightenment, combined with economic necessity, strategic concerns, and scientific curiosity, the various expeditions traversed the Americas and the Pacific Ocean. While the economic benefit to the Spanish Empire is debatable, and perhaps even ran counter to the stated goals of the Bourbon reforms, the role of these explorations as a precursor to the launching of the Philanthropic Expedition was priceless. In addition, many of these undertakings had a clearly medical component to them. Explorers searched for both new diseases and new treatments and provided medical assistance to local populations.

It took the timely collision of a number of catalysts to effect Balmis's great undertaking. Smallpox ravaged the provinces of the Spanish Empire throughout the eighteenth century. Localized outbreaks and epidemics brought in through mercantile activity, the arrival of soldiers, and the slave trade continued to sweep over the American continents. Europe and the colonies experienced hundreds of thousands of deaths from smallpox at this time. The deaths were more than individual human tragedies, however, as they affected the economy and defense of the empire. In an era where a rapid influx of European population was occurring in the American colonies, the growth of New Spain, New Granada, Río de la Plata, and Peru was limited. A disease such as smallpox presented a severe limiting agent to the hopes of Spanish expansionism. Likewise, while diseases such as yellow fever and malaria certainly helped to protect Madrid's interests in the Caribbean by repeatedly decimating English invasion forces, the illnesses also annually reduced the sizes of Spanish garrisons.

The various endeavors known collectively as the Bourbon reforms were launched to address the political, social, economic, technological, and strategic issues confronting the Spanish Empire. While much of this focused around improving and expanding trade, rethinking the defense of the Americas, and reorganizing the government bureaucracy, Charles III and Charles IV also endeavored to expand their scientific knowledge of the New World and address the public health crisis there.

At the same time, local entities also attempted to reform the current state of public health and sanitation in the colonies. Though royally appointed, governors were products of both the Catholic Church and the Enlightenment, and many sought to use their positions for the improvement of the population. In the half century leading up to the launching of the Balmis Expedition, numerous hospitals were constructed in major cities, medical schools were established or expanded, cemeteries specifically designed for victims of contagion were laid out, new regulations were enforced, and variolation was even encouraged. The last was a particularly debated method of preventing epidemic outbreaks of smallpox, and while generally supported by the Catholic Church, the process was still mistrusted or even despised by a percentage of the population.

Finally, the personal health concerns of the Bourbon rulers themselves certainly played a role in the decision to launch the expedition. The destruction wrought by smallpox as well as other diseases on the royal family threatened to weaken their hold on power. The early death of Louis I stands out as a particular example, while Charles IV lost numerous siblings to the scourge of pestilence. Likewise, though Charles IV eagerly embraced the practice of variolation to counter this threat, its shortcomings left him open to accepting a safer and more reliable method.

Thus, Spain was well placed to receive Edward Jenner's gift at the close of the eighteenth century. Far from the medically backward nation it was later portrayed to be by the English and others, Spain was still very much at the forefront of science, empire building, and culture at the time. The early translation and rapid dissemination of works by Jenner, Moreau, and others demonstrate this. The fact that similar schemes on a smaller scale were being proposed or carried out by various other nations proves that

Spain was still very much in line with contemporaneous public health efforts.

The planning for and launching of the Balmis Expedition was a marvel of logistical effort. Considering the current threats and dangers of the Napoleonic Wars, the expedition was both a public health coup and, perhaps, a demonstration of Spain's confidence in its security. Overall, the expedition's organization was a credit to the administrative reforms carried out by the Bourbons. The focus on selecting persons who had firsthand knowledge of the landscape and bureaucracy present in the colonies was an important decision at a time when most great undertakings in Europe were assigned to favorites or used as political rewards. Even the selection of orphans as carriers for the virus was done in a scientific and humanitarian way.

Yet the Balmis Expedition came into conflict with several historical processes. The development of society in Latin America had reached a stage comparable to that of the English colonies in the 1760s. A quest by the landed elites for more political power and a desire by others to assert themselves as equal in status to those in the Iberian Peninsula caused any direct intervention by Madrid to be seen as yet another example of stifling direct rule. The efforts by even royally appointed governors to acquire vaccine material ahead of the arrival of Balmis and Salvany, or else to limit their activities, were perhaps to bolster their own standing in the rapidly changing power structure in the colonies.

The advance of Napoleon in Europe also meant the subsequent destabilization and downfall of the Spanish monarchy. The historical revisionism that followed this event did much to discredit the previous accomplishments of the Bourbons. A political revolution in Spain needed to establish the former regime as incompetent and evil. This development broadened the already present Black Legend and led to the narrative's adoption by many in Spain. Thus, only a few years after the return of the expedition, the memory of it quickly faded from the public record or was painted in darker terms as a financial waste, an example of absolutism and imperial overreach, or a misapplication of resources during a time of imminent invasion.

The long-term accomplishments of Balmis and his expedition are now becoming more recognized and rest on two general achievements. The first is purely humanitarian and demographic, in that hundreds of thousands of people were directly vaccinated. Many of these were subsequently spared infection or death from smallpox. Any reduction of the number of people susceptible to infection would have dramatically lowered the risks of the disease turning epidemic. The tens of thousands or more who avoided being killed by smallpox were thereafter able to participate in the economy and society as well as to have children. The impact Balmis, Salvany, and Charles IV had on Latin America and the Philippines was enormous.

The second long-term accomplishment of the humanitarian voyage was as a model for subsequent attempts at large-scale government efforts to improve public health. Though improving the health and well-being of the population has long been a hallmark of benevolent leaders throughout history, the rise of modern science and medicine, the advent of absolutism, and the demands of democracy have all led to public health becoming a pronounced cornerstone of modern rule. All of these things combined for perhaps the first time in the launching of the Balmis Expedition. Subsequent attempts by various governments to conduct similar undertakings owe their start to Charles IV and the physicians of the voyage.

Perhaps the most influential aspect of Balmis's efforts was his attempt to spread the vaccine to China and Saint Helena. While the move by Charles IV to inoculate his own population may be written off by economic or political motives as much as by humanitarian concerns, Balmis's push to spread the material to both China and to the British during a time of war stands out in the annals of public medicine. The advance of science in the sixteenth to eighteenth centuries had given rise to the knowledge that disease not only affected the poor in a society but also quickly spread to the elite and rulers. Thus efforts were undertaken to improve the sanitation and public health of early modern countries to benefit the rulers as much as to benefit the ruled. Balmis's efforts evolved this proposition to the next stage. Disease did not recognize socioeconomic or national boundaries. While the Spanish doctor's efforts may have been altruistic, it soon became apparent to many as the nineteenth century wore on that battling disease in these distant lands was more and more necessary to prevent illness from reaching Europe and North America. As the twentieth century progressed, international efforts to confront polio, malaria, smallpox, and COVID-19 did exactly that.

Recently, former president Jimmy Carter's campaign to eliminate Guinea worm infections in Africa is a good example of a purely altruistic effort to combat disease in other countries. George W. Bush's organization of PEPFAR, which did much to help lower the rate of AIDS in sub-Saharan Africa, is another application of Flores's and Balmis's ideas. While Bush's announcement in 2003 that he was calling for $15 billion to help combat the disease in Africa was met by both surprise and acclaim, the program was not without its critics. Much as with Spanish efforts in the Americas, claims of scientific absolutism were soon hurled at the administration.[2] This largely centered around the program's focus on abstinence education, which consumed upward of one-third of the funding. Critics lambasted what they saw as attempts to push outside morality onto local cultures, with little demonstrable results.[3] Opponents of the president saw the focus on abstinence education as stemming from his Christian ideology and from his discrediting of local traditional cultural ideas.[4] Like much of the criticism leveled at Balmis, this critique of method had more to do with politics and a misunderstanding of cultural similarities than it did with actual absolutism. Much of this region tended to be religiously and socially conservative, and abstinence was not unknown in the area. As one researcher wrote, "The debate over 'what happened in Uganda' continues, often involving divisive abstinence-versus-condoms rhetoric, which appears more related to the culture wars in the USA than to African social reality."[5]

The Balmis Expedition was a culmination of centuries of Spanish history, local societal trends, church efforts, medical advancements, and the clash of the Enlightenment and absolutism. As the French Revolution was collapsing and Napoleon was pushing forward on all fronts, King Charles IV of Spain sent out a ship that was to save the lives of hundreds of thousands of people. This great philanthropic undertaking ushered in two centuries of worldwide attempts to eliminate disease as a threat to humanity. Balmis and Salvany's journey was not without conflict or consequence, as it served as a social, political, medical, and economic change agent for Latin America and the world. In effect, the Philanthropic Expedition represented the last action of the Spanish Empire and the first undertaking of the modern medical establishment.

Notes

INTRODUCTION

1. "Smallpox Virus Escapes: Tragedy Trails Lab's Error," *Lawrence Journal World*, March 4, 1979, 6B.
2. Campbell Docherty, "Toxic Shock," *Birmingham Post*, October 4, 2003.
3. Benjamin Valentino, *Final Solutions: Mass Killing and Genocide in the 20th Century* (Ithaca: Cornell University Press, 2005), 75, 91, and 275.
4. Anthony S. Fauci and Robert W. Eisinger, "PEPFAR-15 Years and Counting the Lives Saved," *New England Journal of Medicine* 378, no. 4 (2018): 314–16.

CHAPTER I

1. William Rosen, *Justinian's Flea: Plague, Empire, and the Birth of Europe* (New York: Viking Adult, 2007), 3.
2. Sergio Sabbatani, Roberto Manfredi, and Sirio Fiorino, "The Justinian Plague: Influence of the Epidemic on the Rise of the Islamic Empire," *Le Infezioni in Medicina* 20, no. 3 (September 2012): 217–32; Michael W. Dols, "Plague in Early Islamic History," *Journal of the American Oriental Society* 94, no. 3 (July–September, 1974): 371–83.
3. Quoted in William Jackson, *The Rock of the Gibraltarians* (Cranbury, N.J.: Associated University Presses, 1986), 52.
4. Robert Hughes, *Barcelona* (New York: Vintage, 1993), 142.
5. Joseph Patrick Byrne, *Encyclopedia of the Black Death*, vol. 1 (Santa Barbara: ABC CLIO, 2012), 31.
6. Hughes, *Barcelona*, 142–43.
7. "The Work of the Holy Name Society in America," *Ecclesiastical Review*, vol. 44 (Philadelphia: Dolphin, 1911), 642–43.
8. Margarita Cabrera Sanchez, "La epidemia de 1488 en Córdoba," *Anuario de estudios medievales* 39, no. 1 (2009): 223–44.
9. Joseph Patrick Byrne, *The Black Death* (Westport, Conn.: Greenwood, 2004), 111.
10. W. B. Ober, "The Plague at Granada, 1348–1349: Ibn al-Khatib and the Ideas of Contagion," *Bulletin of the NY Academy of Medicine* 58, no. 4 (May 1982): 418–24.
11. *Sahih al-Bukhari*, vol. 4, book 52, number 82–83, states that "Allah's Apostle said, 'Five are regarded as martyrs: They are those who die because of plague, abdominal disease, drowning or a falling building etc., and the martyrs in Allah's Cause'" and, "The Prophet said, 'Plague is the cause of martyrdom of every Muslim (who dies because of it).'"
12. Meredith Hindley, "The Spanish Ulcer," *Humanities* 31, no. 1 (January/February 2010).

13. Solomon ibn Verga, *Shevet Yehudah*, quoted in Yosef H. Yerushalmi, *The Lisbon Massacre of 1506 and the Royal Image in the Shebet Yehudah* (Cincinnati: Hebrew Union College, 1976), 2.

14. W. Schreiber, *Infectio* (Basel: Editione Roche, 1987), 8.

15. James D. Tracy, *Emperor Charles V, Impresario of War: Campaign, Strategy, International Finance, and Domestic Policies* (Cambridge: Cambridge University Press, 2002), 35.

16. Ruy Diaz de Isla, *Serpentine Malady* (1539).

17. See M. Healy, *Fictions of Disease in Early Modern England: Bodies, Plagues and Politics* (New York: Springer, 2001).

18. Peter Pierson, *Commander of the Armada: The Seventh Duke of Medina Sidonia* (New Haven: Yale University Press, 1989), 82–83.

19. Duke of Medina-Sidona, *Letter to the King of Spain, Philip II* (June 24, 1588). English sources report that after the capture of the *Nuestra Senora del Rosario*, its bread was found to be "full of worms."

20. Michael Lewis, *The Spanish Armada* (New York: Pan Books, 1960), 179.

21. Letter, Medina-Sidonia to King Philip II (September 1588).

22. Diary of Juan de Saavedra (September 23, 1588).

23. Letter, Lord Howard to William Cecil (August 20, 1588).

24. As quoted in Peter Whitefield, *Sir Francis Drake* (London: British Library, 2004), 133.

25. Whitefield, 136.

26. Enrique Laval, "El Garotillo en España (Siglos XVI y XVII)," *Chilean Journal of Infectology* 23, no. 1 (March 2006): 78–80.

27. Pavon Magonto, "Henry IV of Castilla (1454–1474): An Exceptional Urologic Patient. An Endocrinopathy Causing the Uro-Andrological Problems of the Monarch. Artificial Insemination Attempts (IV)," *Archivos espanoles de urologia* 56, no. 3 (2003): 222–32.

28. "Diseases and Causes of Death Among the Popes," *Acta Theologica Supplementum* 7 (2005): 240.

29. Maria Gomez, *Juana of Castile: History and Myth of the Mad Queen* (Lewisburg: Bucknell University Press, 2008), 35.

30. See Gomez, *Juana of Castile* and Bethany Aram, "Juana 'the Mad's' Signature: The Problem of Invoking Royal Authority, 1505–1507," *Sixteenth Century Journal* 29, no. 2 (Summer 1998): 331–58.

31. Tracy, *Emperor Charles V*, 239.

32. J. de Zulueta, "The Cause of Death of Emperor Charles V," *Parassitologia* 49, nos. 1–2 (June 2007): 107–9.

33. Catrina Whitley, "A New Explanation for the Reproductive Woes and Midlife Decline of Henry VIII," *Cambridge Historical Journal* 53, no. 4 (December 2010): 827–48.

34. Ewen Callaway, "Inbred Royals Show Traces of Natural Selection," *Nature* (April 19, 2013).

35. Philip Van Kerrebroeck, "Urological Problems in Spanish Royalty" (lecture, Urological Conference, Madrid, March 21, 2015).
36. Igor Babkin, "The Origin of the Variola Virus," *Viruses* 7, no. 3 (March 2015): 1100–1112.
37. Ana T. Duggan, Maria F. Perdomo, Dario Piombino-Mascali, Stephanie Marciniak, Debi Poinar, Matthew V. Emery, Jan P. Buchmann, et al. "17th Century Variola Virus Reveals the Recent History of Smallpox," *Current Biology* 26, no. 24 (2016): 3407–12.
38. James C. Moore, *The History of Smallpox* (London: Longman, 1815), 77.
39. Robert McCaa, "Spanish and Nahuatl Views on Smallpox and Demographic Catastrophe in Mexico," *Journal of Interdisciplinary Studies* 25, no. 3 (Winter 1995): 417.
40. McCaa, "Views on Smallpox," 418.
41. Moore, *History of Smallpox*, 96.

CHAPTER 2

1. Jordi Gómez i Prat and Sheila Mendonça de Souza have done much research on the presence of tuberculosis in North and South America before the arrival of the Spanish. In some cases, outbreaks of the disease reached epidemic scale in isolated settings because of a variety of population stresses and outside factors. These include over 133 confirmed cases stretching back almost two thousand years.
2. McCaa, "Views on Smallpox," 424.
3. Bernal Díaz del Castillo, Janet Burke, and Ted Humphrey, *The True History of the Conquest of New Spain* (Indianapolis: Hackett, 2012), 434.
4. *Cocoliztli* is the Nahuatl world for "plague" or "pestilence."
5. Rodolfo Acuna-Soto, Leticia Calderon Romero, and James H. Maguire, "Large Epidemics of Hemorrhagic Fevers in Mexico, 1545–1815," *American Journal of Tropical Medicine and Hygiene* 62 (2000): 733–39.
6. Acuna-Soto, Calderon Romero, and Maguire, 733–39.
7. Sarah Gibbens, "What Wiped Out the Aztecs? Scientists Find New Clues," *National Geographic*, January 16, 2018.
8. The corresponding endnote citation is: Acuna-Soto, R., et al., "Megadrought and Megadeath in 16th Century Mexico," *Emerging Infectious Diseases*, Vol. 8, Issue 4 (2002): 360-362
9. Guamán Poma de Ayala Felipe and Christopher Dilke, *Letter to a King: A Peruvian Chief's Account of Life Under the Incas and Under Spanish Rule* (New York: Dutton, 1978).
10. For a discussion of the various diseases that are held responsible for the death of Huayna Capac and others, see Robert McCaa, Aleta Nimlos, and Teodoro Hampe-Martinez, "Why Blame Smallpox? The Death of the Inca Huayna Capac and the Demographic Destruction of Tawantinsuyu" (American Historical Association Annual Meeting, January 8–11, 2004).
11. McCaa, Nimlos, and Hampe-Martinez, "Why Blame Smallpox?" Carlos Sempat Assadourian does much to discount traditional notions of the fall of the Inca in "La

gran vejación y destruición de la tierra: Las guerras de sucesión y de conquista en el derrumbe de la población indígena del Perú," in *Transiciones hacia el sistema colonial andino* (Lima: Instituto de Estudios Peruanos, 1994), 19–62.

12. R. C. Robertson, *Rotting Face: Smallpox and the American Indian* (Caldwell: Cauton, 2001), 52.

13. James Mooney, "Sacred Formula of the Cherokee," in *Seventh Annual Report of the Bureau of Ethnology to the Secretary of the Smithsonian Institution 1885-'86*, ed. John Wesley Powell, Walter James Hoffman, and James Mooney (Washington, D.C.: Smithsonian Institution and GPO, 1891), 337.

14. Cabeza de Vaca, *Chronicles of the Narvaez Expedition* (New York: W. W. Norton, 2013), 35–36. Thomas Harriot reported a similar practice in his *Brief and True Report of the New Found Land of Virginia* (Elizabeth City, N.C.: Michael R. Worthington, 2017). Also see Henry Spelman, *Relation of Virginia* (London: Chiswick, 1872), 40.

15. Charles H. Townshend, "The Quinnipiack Indians and Their Reservation," in *Papers of the New Haven Colonial Historical Society*, vol. 6 (New Haven, Conn.: New Haven Colonial Historical Society Press, 1900), 156.

16. August Hirsch and Charles Creighton, *Handbook of Geographical and Historical Pathology,* vol. 1 (London: New Sydenham Society, 1883), 136.

17. Donald R. Hopkins, *Smallpox: The Greatest Killer in History* (Chicago: University of Chicago Press, 1983), 205.

18. Hopkins, 205.

19. Hopkins, 213.

20. Sebastián Lorente, *Historia del Perú bajo la dinastia austriaca 1542–1598*, vol. 1 (Lima: B. Gil, 1863), 357.

21. Hopkins, *Smallpox*, 214.

22. Hopkins, 215.

23. N. A. M. Rodger, *The Command of the Ocean: A Naval History of Britain* (New York: W. W. Norton, 2004), 308.

24. Jonathan R. Dull, *The Age of the Ship of the Line: The British and French Navies, 1650–1815* (Lincoln: University of Nebraska Press, 2009), 46.

25. Thomas Philip Terry, *Terry's Mexico* (London: Gay and Hancock, 1911), 396–97.

26. Mary Ellen Snodgrass, *World Epidemics: A Cultural Chronology of Disease* (Jefferson, N.C.: McFarland, 2017), 101.

27. Martha Few, "Circulating Smallpox Knowledge: Guatemalan Doctors, Maya Indians and Designing Spain's Smallpox Vaccination Expedition," *British Journal for the History of Science* 43, no. 4 (December 2010): 521.

28. Moore, *History of Smallpox*, 287–88.

29. James E. McClellan III, *Colonialism and Science: Saint Domingue and the Old Regime* (Chicago: University of Chicago Press, 2010), 1144.

CHAPTER 3

1. *Mozi*, Book 7, "Will of Heaven," III, 3.

2. Lev. 12:2 (New King James Version).

3. Num. 16:47–48 (NKJV).

4. 2 Sam. 24:15–17 (NKJV).

5. Mark 16:17–18 (NKJV).

6. Acts 3:6–7 (NKJV).

7. Matt. 10:8 (NKJV).

8. *The Rule of St. Benedict,* chapter 36, traditionalcatholic.net/Tradition/Information/Saint/Benedict/The_Holy_Rule/Chapter-36.html.

9. Ulrich Lehner, *The Catholic Enlightenment: The Forgotten History of a Global Movement* (Oxford: Oxford University Press, 2016), 20.

10. William of Malmesbury, *Chronicle* (London: Henry G. Bohn, 1847), 246–47.

11. *Cantigas de Santa Maria,* number 321, lines 30–33.

12. *Cantigas,* line 45.

13. See Joseph O'Callaghan, *Alfonso X and the Cantigas de Santa Maria: A Poetic Biography* (Leiden: Brill, 1988), 76–80.

14. Thomas Hobbes, *Leviathan,* bk. 2, chapter 29.

15. Thomas More, *Utopia,* bk. 2.

16. Baron de Montesquieu, *The Spirit of Laws,* bk. 14, chapter 11.

17. Montesquieu, bk. 14, chapter 11.

18. Montesquieu, bk. 23, chapter 29.

19. Moore, *History of Smallpox,* 287–88.

20. Arnold of Villanova, *Liber de Vinis,* trans. Wilhelm von Hirnkofen (New York: Harper, 1943), 24.

21. Roger Bigelow Merriman, "The Cortes of the Spanish Kingdoms in the Later Middle Ages," *American Historical Review* 16, no. 3 (April 1911): 476–95.

22. John Lynch, *Bourbon Spain* (Oxford: Basil Blackwell, 1989), 156.

23. Allan Kuethe, *The Spanish Atlantic World in the Eighteenth Century: War and the Bourbon Reforms* (Cambridge: Cambridge University Press, 2014), 7.

CHAPTER 4

1. For a discussion of the cost of the expedition, see Victor W. Von Hagen, "Francisco Hernandez: Naturalist," *Scientific Monthly* 58, no. 5 (May 1944): 383–85.

2. Francisco Hernández to Philip II, November/December 1571, in *The Mexican Treasury: The Writings of Dr. Francisco Hernández,* ed. Simon Varey, trans. Rafael Chabrán, Cynthia L Chamberlin, and Simon Varey (Stanford: Stanford University Press, 2000), 48–49.

3. Varey, 48–49.

4. Donatella Lippi, "Chocolate in History: Food, Medicine, Medi-food," *Nutrients* 5, no. 5 (May 2013): 1573–84.

5. Francisco Hernández to Philip II, April 30, 1572, in Varey, *Writings of Dr. Francisco Hernández,* 49–50.

6. Varey, 49–50.

7. Martyn Rix, *The Golden Age of Botanical Art* (Chicago: University of Chicago Press, 2012), 118.

8. Eric J. Tepe, "A Series of Unfortunate Events: The Forgotten Botanist and the Misattribution of a Type Collection," *PhytoKeys* 109 (2018): 33–39.

9. José Ramón Marcaida and Juan Pimentel, "Green Treasures and Paper Floras: The Business of Mutis in New Granada (1783–1808)," *History of Science* 52, no. 3 (September 2014): 277–96.

10. First published in 2010 as Edward O. Wilson, *Kingdom of Ants: José Celestino Mutis and the Dawn of Natural History in the New World* (Baltimore: Johns Hopkins University Press, 2010).

11. Daniela Bleichmer, *Visible Empire: Botanical Expeditions and Visual Culture in the Hispanic Enlightenment* (Chicago: University of Chicago, 2012), 142.

12. Bleichmer, 125.

13. Felipe Fernández-Armesto, *Pathfinders: A Global History of Exploration* (New York: W. W. Norton, 2006), 305–7.

14. Jonathan Lamb, "Captain Cook and the Scourge of Scurvy," BBC, History, February 17, 2011.

15. Christopher R. Boyer, *A Land Between Waters: Environmental Histories of Modern Mexico* (Tucson: University of Arizona Press, 2012), 74.

16. Bleichmer, *Visible Empire*, 142.

17. José Mariano Moziño and Iris Wilson Engstrand, *Noticias de Nutka: An Account of Nootka Sound in 1792* (Seattle: University of Washington Press, 1991), xxv.

CHAPTER 5

1. Francis Darwin, "Francis Galton," *The Eugenics Review*, Vol. 6, Issue 1 (1914), 1.

2. Stefan Riedal, "Edward Jenner and the History of Smallpox and Vaccination," *Baylor University Medical Center Proceedings* 18, no. 11 (January 2005): 21–25.

3. Patrick J. Pead, "Benjamin Jesty: New Light in the Dawn of Vaccination," *Lancet* 362, no. 9401 (December 20–27, 2003): 2104–9.

4. George Pearson, *An Inquiry Concerning the History of the Cowpox* (London: J Johnson, 1798), 84–85.

5. Arthur Bolyston, "The Myth of the Milkmaid," *New England Journal of Medicine* 378, no. 5 (February 1, 2018): 414–15.

6. Jason Tetro, *The Germ Code* (Toronto: Doubleday Canada, 2013), 35.

7. Thomas Dudley Fosbroke, *Berkeley Manuscripts* (London: John Nichols and Son, 1821), 221–22.

8. F. Dawtry Drewitt, *The Life of Edward Jenner* (Cambridge: Cambridge University Press, 2013), 62.

9. José G. Rigau-Pérez, "The Introduction of Smallpox Vaccine in 1803 and the Adoption of Immunization as a Government Function in Puerto Rico," *Hispanic American Historical Review* 69, no. 3 (August 1989): 394.

10. "Miscellany," *Medical Record* 95 (May 3, 1919), 760.

11. Gilabert seems to have later served on the junta that was established in the region in 1812 during the Napoleonic Wars. María Pilar Hernando Serra, *El ayunta-*

miento de Valencia y la invasión napoleónica (Valéncia: Universitat de Valéncia, 2004), 153.

12. "Galeria de Alicantinos Ilustres," *El Archivo*, vol. 2 (Denia: Imprenta de Pedro Botella, 1887), 158.

13. "Galeria de Alicantinos Ilustres," 158.

14. Michele Clouse, *Medicine, Government and Public Health in Philip II's Spain* (London: Routledge, 2016), 7.

15. Fiona Clark, *Ireland and Medicine in the 17th and 18th Centuries* (Farnham: Ashgate, 2010), 206.

16. As quoted in Gonzalo Díaz de Yraola, *La vuelta al mundo de la expedición de la vacuna (1803–1810)* (Madrid: CSIC, 2003), 25.

17. Fiona Clark, "Appealing to the Republic of Letters: An Autopsy of Anti-venereal Trials in Eighteenth-Century Mexico," *Social History of Medicine* 27, no. 1 (February 2014): 2–21.

18. De Yraola, *Expedición de la vacuna*, 26.

19. "Galeria de Alicantinos Ilustres," 161.

20. Clark, "Republic of Letters," 11.

21. Alexander von Humboldt, *Personal Narrative of Travels to the Equinoctial Regions of America During the Years 1799–1804*, vol. 1 (Covent Gardens: George Bell and Sons, 1889), 381.

22. Rigau-Pérez, "Introduction of Smallpox Vaccine," 394.

23. Jacques-Louis Moreau de La Sarthe, *Traité historique et pratique de la vaccine* (Paris: Editions Champion-Slatkine, 1801), v.

24. José Tuells, "The Revision Process of Francisco Xavier Balmis' Translation of Moreau de La Sarthe's Historical and Practical Treatise on Vaccines," *Gaceta Sanitaria* 26, no. 4 (July–August 2012): 372–75.

CHAPTER 6

1. Martha E. Rodriguez, "Articulating Medical Ideas: Medicine and Medical Education in New Spain," in *Biomedicine as a Contested Site: Some Revelations in Imperial Contexts*, ed. Poonam Bala (Plymouth: Lexington, 2009), 140.

2. Marcus Cueto, *Medicine and Public Health in Latin America* (Cambridge: Cambridge University Press, 2015), 48.

3. Donald B. Cooper, *Epidemic Disease in Mexico City, 1761–1813* (Austin: University of Texas Press, 2015), 62.

4. Cooper, 66.

5. Robin Price, "State Church Charity and Smallpox: An Epidemic Crisis in the City of Mexico, 1797–1798," *Journal of the Royal Society of Medicine* 75, no. 5 (May 1982): 361.

6. Based on the near-contemporaneous estimates of Cosme de Mier y Trespalacios.

7. Price, "State Church Charity," 356.

8. Domingo Cabello to Teodoro de Croix (November 20, 1780), Bexar Archives, Box 2C44, L.S., pp. 1–2v.

9. Domingo Cabello to Jacobo de Ugarto y Loyola (November 5, 1786), Bexar Archives, Box 2C61, Df.S, pp. i–iv.

10. Domingo Cabello to Cabildo (November 9, 1786), Bexar Archives, Box 2C61, L.S., pp. i–iv and Domingo Cabello to Luis Cazorla (November 6, 1786), Bexar Archives, Box 2C61, L.S., pp. i.

11. Price, "State Church Charity," 362–63.

12. Price, 364–65.

13. For a full accounting of this figure, see Cooper, *Epidemic Disease.*

14. Price, "State Church Charity," 367.

15. Archivo General de Centro America A1.4.7-4026.31004 (September 5, 1780).

16. Few, "Circulating Smallpox Knowledge," 525.

17. José Flores, *Instrucción sobre el modo de practicar la inoculación de las viruelas, y el mótodo para curar esta enfermedad acomodado a la naturaleza y modo de vivir los Indios del reyno de Guatemala* (Nueva Guatemala: Ignacio Beteta, 1793), 3.

18. José Flores, "Report to the Council of the Indies," as quoted in de Yraola, *Expedición de la vacuna,* 39.

19. Quoted in Few, "Circulating Smallpox Knowledge," 532.

20. Pedro Lautaro Ferrer, *Historia general de la medicina en Chile* (Talca: Impr. Talca de J. Martin Garrido C, 1904), 132–33.

21. Paul Ramirez, "'Like Herod's Massacre': Quarantines, Bourbon Reform, and Popular Protest in Oaxaca's Smallpox Epidemic, 1796–1797," *The Americas* 69, no. 2 (October 2010): 203–I.

22. Allyson M. Poska, "Public Health, Peasant Bodies and the Spanish Colonisation of Patagonia," *Social History of Medicine* 25, no. 2 (2011): 290–306.

23. Robert J. Ferry, *The Colonial Elite of Early Caracas: Formation and Crisis, 1567–1767* (Berkeley: University of California Press, 1989), 226.

24. For more information on the role that disease in general played in reform movements in New Granada, see Emilio Quevado, *Historia de la medicina en Colombia: De la medicina ilustrada a la medicina anatomoclínica (1782–1865)* (Bogotá: Tecnoquímicas, 2007).

25. Richard Slatta, *Simón Bolívar's Quest for Glory* (College Station: Texas A&M Press, 2003), 81.

26. Hopkins, *Smallpox,* 44.

27. Henry Karmen, *Philip V of Spain: The King Who Reigned Twice* (New Haven, Conn.: Yale University Press, 2001), 150.

28. Elizabeth King, "Clockwork Prayer: A Sixteenth-Century Mechanical Monk," *Blackbird* 1, no. 1 (Spring 2002).

29. Robert McCaa, "The Peopling of Mexico," in *A Population History of North America,* ed. Michael R. Haines (Cambridge: Cambridge University Press, 2000), 260.

30. Nicolau Barquet and Pere Domingo, "Smallpox: The Triumph over the Most Terrible of the Ministers of Death," *Annals of Internal Medicine* 127, no. 8 (1999): 635–42.

31. John Wilton Appel, "Francisco José de Caldas: A Scientist at Work in Nueva Granada," *Transactions of the American Philosophical Society* 84, part 5 (1994): 22.

32. Jane Landers, *Slavery and Abolition in the Atlantic World: New Sources and New Findings* (New York: Taylor and Francis, 2017), 40–58.

33. Frank Safford, *The Ideal of the Practical: Colombia's Struggle to Form a Technical Elite* (Austin: University of Texas Press, 1976), chap. 4, 34n.

34. Esparragosa did much to elevate the field of medical arts in Guatemala and invented a new standard of forceps to aid in the delivery of infants.

35. Christopher T. Leffler and Ricardo Wainsztein, "The First Cataract Surgeons in Latin America: 1611–1830," *Clinical Ophthalmology* 10 (2016): 679–94.

36. Archivo General de Indias, Indiferente General 1558H, Carta de Jose Flores al Consejo de Indias (February 28, 1803).

37. Excerpted in de Yraola, *Expedición de la vacuna*, 68.

38. Manuel de Mendiburu, *Historical Biographical Dictionary* (Lima: Solis, 1879), 290.

39. Quoted in A. Ruiz Moreno, *Introduccion de la vacuna en America* (Buenos Aires: Universidad de Buenos Aires, 1947), 18.

40. Manuel de Godoy, *Memorias* (Alicante: Universidad de Alicante, 2008), 919, 1196–98.

41. A. Ruiz Moreno, *Introducción de la vacuna en América (Expedición de Balmis)* (Buenos Aires: Universidad de Buenos Aires, 1947) 18–20. Requena served as the main commissioner in settling the Maynas Province border dispute between Ecuador and Peru as well as in several other boundary disputes.

42. "Sketch of the Progress of Medicine," *Medical and Physical Journal* 26, no. 149 (July–December 1811), 26 and *Monthly Review* 75 (1786), 534.

43. Few, "Circulating Smallpox Knowledge," 520.

44. Archivo General de Indias, Indiferente General 1558H, Carta de Jose Flores al Consejo de Indias (February 28, 1803).

45. Archivo General de Indias.

46. Archivo General de Indias.

47. Abbas Behbehani, "The Smallpox Story: Life and Death of an Old Disease," *Microbiological Reviews* 47, no. 4 (December 1983), 477.

48. Gabriel Moreno, *Almanac and Guide for Outsiders* (Lima, 1907).

49. José Tuells and José Luis Duro Torrijo, "El viaje de la vacuna contra la viruela: Una expedición, dos océanos, tres continentes, y miles de niños," *Gazeta Medica de Mexico* 151, no. 3 (2015): 416–25.

CHAPTER 7

1. *Gazeta de Madrid*, no. 62 (August 5, 1803), 676.

2. De Yraola, *Expedición de la vacuna*, 43.

3. Michael M. Smith, "Royal Vaccination Expeditions," *American Philosophical Society* 64, no. 1 (1974) 1–74.

4. *Diario de las discusiones y actas de las Cortes*, vol. 18 (Cádiz: La Imprenta Nacional, 1813), 26.

5. Archivo General de Indias, Indiferente General 1558H, Carta de Jose Flores al Consejo de Indias (November 5, 1803).

6. Rigau-Pérez, "Introduction of Smallpox Vaccine," 396.

7. F. Balmis, "18 junio 1803, Enterado de su nombramiento." En Diaz de Iraola, G., "La vuelta al mundo de la expedicion de la vacuna," *Anuario de Estudios Americanos*, vol. 4 (1947), 234.

8. Quoted in Antonio Lopez Mariño, *Isabel Zendal Gomez en los Archivos de Galicia* (Parlamento de Galicia, 2018), 34.

9. Jorge Bustos, *Vida Cipotudas: Momentos Estelares Del Empecinamiento Español* (Madrid: La Esfera de los Libros, 2018), 126.

10. The last of these, Benito Vélez, was the child of Isabel Zendal and lived with her in Mexico after the end of the expedition.

11. Expositos enviados a la Expedicion de la Vacuna (1803), Archivo de la Universidad de Santiago de Compostela. Fondo Hospital de los Reyes Catolicos, serie general, no. 785, leg. 20.

12. *Gazeta de Madrid*, no. 104 (December 1, 1803), 1109–14.

13. *Gazeta de Madrid*, no. 6 (January 20, 1804), 57.

14. *Gazeta de Madrid*, no. 6, 49.

15. A. Bethencourt, "Inoculation and Smallpox Vaccine in the Canary Islands (1760–1830)," in *Fifth Colloquium of Canadian-American History*, ed. F. Morales (1982), 280–307.

16. Archivo General de Indias, 2323A, #30, Carta de Francisco Balmis al Jose Antonio Caballero (February 27, 1804).

17. Rigau-Pérez, "Introduction of Smallpox Vaccine," 421.

18. Niklas Thode Jensen, "Safeguarding Slaves: Smallpox, Vaccination, and Governmental Health Policies Among the Enslaved Population in the Danish West Indies, 1803–1848," *Bulletin of the History of Medicine* 83, no. 1 (Spring 2009): 100.

19. Carlos Quiros, "The Smallpox in Peru and Its Eradication: A Historical Account," *Peruvian Journal of Epidemiology* 9, no. 1 (January 1996).

20. Archivo General de Puerto Rico, 124, 1a, Carta Ramon de Castro al Cabildo (February 10, 1804).

21. Archivo General de Indias, 2323A, #30.

22. "Expediente 12," *Extracto General of Expedición philanthropic of vacuna* (Archivo General of Indias. Sección: Indiferente General) Legajo 1558-A.

23. Archivo General de Indias, 2323A, #30.

24. Archivo General de Indias, 2323A, #30.

25. Archivo General de Indias, 2323A, #30.

26. Archivo General de Indias, 2322, #30, "Manifesto de las astenciones politicas que ha observado el Capitan General de Puerto Rico Don Ramon de Castro . . . y desatenciones de Balmis acia el General."

27. Rigau-Perez, "Introduction of Smallpox Vaccine," 415.

28. Archivo General de Puerto Rico, Gobernadores espanoles, caja 121. Carte Toribio Montes al Caballero (December 31, 1804).

29. De Yraola, *Expedición de la vacuna*, 47.

30. Jedidiah Morse, *A New Universal Gazetteer* (New Haven, Conn.: S. Converse, 1823), 152.

31. Jose Esperaza, "Viral Epidemics in Latin America from the 16th to the 19th Centuries and the Early Days of Virology in the Region," in *Human Virology in Latin America: From Biology to Control*, ed. Juan Ernesto Ludert (New York: Springer, 2017), 7; John Tate Lanning, *The Eighteenth-Century Enlightenment in the University of San Carlos de Guatemala* (Ithaca: Cornell University Press, 1956), 252.

32. Cristobal S. Berry-Cabán, "Cuba's First Smallpox Vaccination Campaign," *International Journal of History and Philosophy of Medicine* 5 (2015): 1–4.

33. Berry-Cabán, 4.

34. Adam Warren, *Medicine and Politics in Colonial Peru* (Pittsburgh: University of Pittsburgh Press, 2010), 94.

35. Quoted in Martha Few, *For All of Humanity: Mesoamerican and Colonial Medicine in Enlightenment Guatemala* (Tucson: University of Arizona Press, 2015), 12.

36. Few, *For All of Humanity*, 180; Leffler and Wainsztein, "The First Cataract Surgeons," 679–94.

37. *Gazeta de Mexico* (June 26, 1804).

38. Christon Archer, "Pardos, Indians, and the Army of New Spain: Inter-relationships and Conflict, 1780–1810," *Journal of Latin American Studies* 6, no. 2 (November 1974): 241.

39. Though Hubert Howe Bancroft suggests that Arboleya had unsuccessfully brought vaccine material with him to New Spain from Europe, this would have been too early in the chronology of the introduction of Jenner's method to Spain. Though the physician was most likely aware of the practice while he was in Iberia, it's doubtful he would have tried to carry it across the Atlantic in 1802 or 1803. Hubert Howe Bancroft, *History of the Pacific States of North America: Mexico, 1804–1824*, vol. 7 (San Francisco: Bancroft, 1885), 27.

40. Myron Echenberg, *Humboldt's Mexico: In the Footsteps of the Illustrious German Scientific Traveller* (Montreal: McGill-Queen's University Press, 2017), 193.

41. De Yraola, *Expedición de la vacuna*, 54–56.

42. *Gazeta de Mexico* (June 26, 1804).

43. *Gazeta de Mexico* (May 26, 1804), 96.

44. Alexander von Humboldt, *Personal Narrative of Travels to the Equinoctial Regions of America During the Years 1799–1804*, vol. 1 (London: George Bell and Sons, 1907), chap. 1.11.

45. Archivo General de Indias, Carta Francisco Balmis al Jose Antonio Caballero (January 4, 1805).

46. Smith, "Royal Vaccination Expeditions," 33.

47. Archivo General de Indias, Carta Francisco Balmis al Jose Antonio Caballero (January 4, 1805).

48. Sherburne F. Cook, "Francisco Xavier Balmis and the Introduction of Vaccination to Latin America: Part II," *Bulletin of the History of Medicine* 12, no. 1 (June 1942): 70–101.

49. James Alexander Robertson, *The Hispanic American Historical Review*, vol. 35 (Williams and Wilkins, 1955), 240.

50. Lesley Byrd Simpson, *Many Mexicos* (Berkeley: University of California Press, 1967), 180.

51. E. Soto Perez de Celis, "The Royal Philanthropic Expedition of the Vaccine: A Landmark in the History of Public Health," *Postgraduate Medical Journal* 87, no. 997 (November 2008): 599.

52. Quoted in Paul F. Ramirez, *Enlightened Immunity* (Stanford: Stanford University Press, 2018), 153.

53. Juan Pablo Salazar Andeu, "Manuel Ignacio Gonzalez del Campillo: El Obispo del Dicurso Antiinsurgente," *Revista Mexicana de Historica del Dereccho* 29 (2002): 104–5.

54. Quoted in de Yraola, *Expedición de la vacuna*, 59.

CHAPTER 8

1. "Jose Salvany al Secretario de Gracia y Justica de India, 1 marzo 1805," 1558A, Indiferente General, AGI.

2. For a full discussion of the story, see Antonio Villanueva Edo, *Los heroes olividados* (Barcelona: Rocaeditorial, 2010), chap. 15.

3. "Jose Salvany al Secretario de Gracia y Justica de India, 1 marzo 1805," 1558A, Indiferente General, AGI.

4. R. Tarrago, "The Balmis-Salvany Smallpox Expedition: The First Public Health Vaccination Campaign in South America," *Perspectives in Health: The Magazine of the Pan American Health Organization* 6 (2001): 27.

5. Warren, *Colonial Peru*, 96.

6. "Jose Salvany al Secretario de Gracia y Justica de India, 1 marzo 1805," 1558A, Indiferente General, AGI.

7. Susana Maria Ramirez Martin, *La mayor hazaña medica de la colonia* (Quito: Abya-Yala, 1999), 388.

8. De Yraola, *Expedición de la vacuna*, 69.

9. R. S. Bray, *Armies of Pestilence: The Impact of Disease upon History* (Cambridge: James Clark, 2004), 128.

10. Andres Rosillo y Meruelo, *Sermon of Feb. 24, 1805* (Bogotá: Bruno Espinosa de los Monteros, 1805), 3.

11. Francesc Asensi Botet, "Fighting Against Smallpox Around the World: The Vaccination Expeditions of Xavier de Balmis (1803–1806) and Josep Salvany (1803–1810)," *Contributions to Science* 8, no. 1 (2012): 99–105.

12. Rodney J. Reynolds, "Spreading the Gospel of the Miracle Cure: Panama's Black Christ," in *Cosmos, God, and Madmen: Frameworks in the Anthropologies of Medicine*, ed. Roland Littlewood (New York: Berghahn, 2016), 30.

13. César Rodríguez, "Andean Studies: New Trends and Library Resources," (papers of the Forty-Fifth Annual Meeting of the Seminar on the Acquisition of Latin American Library Materials, Long Beach, California, May 27–31, 2000), 44.

14. Francisco Javier Eugenio Santa Cruz y Espejo, *Escritos del Francisco Javier Eugenio Santa Cruz y Espejo, Tomo II* (Quito: Imprenta Municipal, 1912), 340–43.

15. Quoted in de Yraola, *Expedición de la vacuna*, 72.
16. "Reglamento para las juntas de vacuna del virrey Amat, 19 junio 1805," 1558 A Indiferente General, AGI.
17. Warren, *Colonial Peru*, 102.
18. "José Salvany a Don Antonio Caballero, Secretario de Estado y del Despacho Universal de Gracia y Justica, 1 octubre 1806," 1558A, Indiferente General, AGI.
19. Warren, *Colonial Peru*, 102–15.
20. Patricia Noble, "Technology, the Environment, and Social Change," (papers of the Thirty-Eighth Annual Meeting of the Seminar on the Acquisition of Latin American Library Materials, vol. 38, Instituto de Bibliotecas de la Universidad de Guadalajara, May 15–20, 1993), 63.
21. José Ramón Jouve Martín, *The Black Doctors of Colonial Lima: Science, Race, and Writing in Colonial and Early Republican Peru* (Montreal: McGill-Queen's University Press, 2014), 60–94.
22. Warren, *Colonial Peru*, 105.
23. Warren, 106.
24. Warren, 116.
25. Warren, 115.
26. Diego Barras Arana, *Historia jeneral de Chile*, vol. 7 (Santiago: Rafael Jover, 1886), 275.
27. Barras Arana, 275 .
28. *British and Foreign Medico-chirurgical Review*, vol. 45, January–April 1870 (London: John Churchill and Sons, 1870), 317.

CHAPTER 9
1. Martin de Rada to Guido de Lavezaris (1574) as quoted in Linda A. Newson, *Conquest and Pestilence in the Early Spanish Philippines* (Honolulu: University of Hawaii Press, 2009), 21.
2. Quoted in F. Fernandez del Castillo, *The Trips of D. Francisco Xavier de Balmis* (Mexico City: Ed. Galas de Mexico, 1960).
3. Jacques Chastenet, *Godoy: Master of Spain* (London: Batchworth, 1953), 132.
4. Michael M. Smith, "The Royal Vaccine Expedition to New Spain and Guatemala," *Transactions of the American Philosophical Society* 64, no. 1 (1974): 1–74.
5. Laurence Monnais, *Global Movements, Local Concerns: Medicine and Health in Southeast Asia* (Honolulu: University of Hawaii Press, 2012), 5.
6. Quoted in de Yraola, *Expedición de la vacuna*, 83.
7. Thomas B. Colvin, "Arms Around the World: The Introduction of Smallpox Vaccine into the Philippines and Macao in 1805," *Revista de Cultura* 18 (2006): 74.
8. Michael Levin, "A Brief History of the Population of Guam from 1710 through 1897," in *Guam History*, vol. 2, ed. Lee Carter (Mangilao: Micronesia Area Resource Center, 1997); J. N. Hays, *The Burden of Disease: Epidemics and Human Responses in Western History* (New Brunswick: Rutgers University Press, 2009), 185.

9. James C. Moore, *The History and Practice of Vaccination* (London: J. Callow, 1817), 269.

10. Emma Helen Blair, *The Philippine Islands, 1493–1898: Relating to China and the Chinese*, vol. 23 (Cleveland: Arthur Clark, 1915), 25.

11. Colvin, "Arms Around the World," 76.

12. Aguilar to Zulaibar, May 7, 1805, AAM, Document D. 90. 60, Folio 34-34b, Box 1.D.10, Libro de Gobierno Ecl (1767–1806), Folder 9, Libro de Oficios (Cartas), Fr. Zulaibar.

13. Zulaibar, May 29, 1805, AAM, Box 1.D.10, Libro de Gobierno Ecl (1767-1806), Folder 9, Libro de Oficios (Cartas), Fr. Zulaibar, File D.9.61, ff.34b-36.

14. Ken De Bevoise, *Agents of the Apocalypse: Epidemic Disease in the Colonial Philippines* (Princeton: Princeton University Press, 1995), 160–63.

15. Nicai de Guzman, "The 'Stranger' in Intramures' Plaza: A Roman Saved the Philippines from a Virus," *Esquire*, July 10, 2018.

16. De Bevoise, *Agents of the Apocalypse*, 103.

17. Moore, *History and Practice of Vaccination*, 270.

18. Ambeth Ocampo, "Carlos IV, Manila, and Smallpox," *Philippine Daily Inquirer*, August 20, 2014.

19. Colvin, "Arms Around the World," 81.

20. Warren Hastings to George III, 1780 in Austin Coates, *Macao and the British* (Hong Kong: Oxford University Press, 1988), 78.

21. Quoted in de Yraola, *Expedición de la vacuna*, 87.

22. Francesc Asensi Botet, "La real expedición filantrópica de la vacuna (Xavier de Balmis/Josep Salvany): 1803–1806," *Revista Chilena de Infectologia* 26, no. 6 (2009): 562–67.

23. *Gazeta de Madrid* (October 14, 1806).

24. Letter, General Archive of the Palace of Madrid. Box 16515. Exp. 2.

25. Not to be confused with the ship captain of the same name who transported the expedition across the Pacific.

26. Letter, General Archive of the Nation of Mexico, Epidemics Section, Exp. 18, Box 6177.

27. Francisco Balmis to Real Audiencia (June 30, 1810), General Archive of the Nation of Mexico. Viceroyalty, Epidemics. Exp. 7. Cash 3916.

CHAPTER 10

1. Lidio Cruz Monclova, *Historia de Puerto Rico, Siglo XIX*, vol. 1 (Rio Piedras, 1952): 125.

2. "Smallpox Case in Puerto Rico," *New York Times*, December 24, 1898.

3. "Compulsory Vaccination in Ponce," *New York Times*, January 31, 1899.

4. "Impressions of San Juan," *New York Times*, March 26, 1900.

5. J. Lopez Sanchez, "Tomas Romay and the Yellow Fever," *Journal of the History of Medicine and Allied Sciences* 6, no. 2 (Spring 1951): 195–208.

6. Ross Danielson, *Cuban Medicine* (New Brunswick: Transaction Books, 1979), 51.

7. Berry-Cabán, "Vaccination Campaign," 4.

8. "Cuba's Sad Sanitary State," *New York Times*, May 6, 1896.

9. "Havana's Clean Condition," *New York Times*, May 12, 1899.

10. Monica Garcia, "Typhoid Fever in Nineteenth-Century Colombia: Between Medical Geography and Bacteriology," *Medical History* 58, no. 1 (2014): 27–45.

11. Simón Bolívar, "Measures for the Protection and Wise Use of the Nation's Forest Resources (July 31, 1829)," in *El Libertador: The Writings of Simón Bolívar*, ed. David Bushnell (Oxford: Oxford University Press, 2003), 199.

12. William F. Sater, "The Politics of Public Health: Smallpox in Chile," *Journal of Latin American Studies* 35, no. 3 (August 2003): 525.

13. Sater, 513.

14. Ann Keith Naum, "A History of the First Fifty Years of the Claretian Apostolate in Chile 1870–1923" (master's thesis, Louisiana State University, 1974), 47.

15. Sater, "Politics of Public Health," 517.

16. Barras Arana, *Historia jeneral de Chile*, 277 fn.

17. De Bevoise, *Agents of the Apocalypse*, 103.

18. "Stamping Out Disease in the Philippines," *New York Times*, June 23, 1902.

19. Fulgencio Carrillo, "Carta Decimaquarta," *El Reganon General* (February 29, 1804), 136.

20. Quoted in *British and Foreign Medico-chirurgical Review*, vol. 44, July–October 1869 (London: John Churchill and Sons, 1869), 335.

21. *British and Foreign Medico-chirurgical Review*, 333–34.

22. Letter, George Washington to William Shippen (January 6, 1777) in *The Papers of George Washington*, Revolutionary War Series, *vol. 8, 6 January 1777–27 March 1777*, ed. Frank E. Grizzard Jr. (Charlottesville: University Press of Virginia, 1998), 264.

23. E. P. Hennock, "Vaccination Policy Against Smallpox, 1835–1914: A Comparison of England with Prussia and Imperial Germany," *Social History of Medicine* 11, no. 1 (April 1998): 49–71.

24. G. R. De Beer, "The Relations Between Fellows of the Royal Society and French Men of Science when France and Britain Were at War," *Notes and Records of the Royal Society of London* 9, no. 2 (May 1952): 297.

25. Alexander Grab, "Smallpox Vaccination in Napoleonic Italy," *Napoleonica. La Revue*, no. 30 (March 2017): 38–58.

26. Byrd S. Leavell, "Thomas Jefferson and Smallpox Vaccination," *Transactions of the American Clinical and Climatological Association* 88 (1977): 119–27.

27. Thomas Jefferson to George C. Jenner (May 14, 1806) in *The Jefferson Papers*, Founders Online, National Archives, founders.archives.gov/documents/Jefferson/99-01-02-3718.

28. Moore, *History and Practice of Vaccination*, 270–71.

29. John Z. Bowers, "The Odyssey of Smallpox Vaccination," *Bulletin of the History of Medicine* 55, no. 1 (1981): 30.

30. John Z. Bowers, "The Warm Chain," *Assignment Child* 69 (1985): 231–33.

31. Dong Shaoxin, "Odes on Guiding Smallpox Out: Qiu Xi's Contributions to Vaccination in China," *Revista de Cultura* 18 (2006): 99–111.

32. Shaoxin, 105.

33. *British and Foreign Medico-chirurgical Review*, vol. 45, 318.

34. *British and Foreign Medico-chirurgical Review*, vol. 45, 322–23.

35. *British and Foreign Medico-chirurgical Review*, vol. 44, 328.

36. *British and Foreign Medico-chirurgical Review*, vol. 45, 321–22.

37. Franco Maria Buonaguro, Maria Lina Tornesello, and Luigi Buonaguro, "The XIX Century Smallpox Prevention in Naples and the Risk of Transmission of Human Blood-Related Pathogens," *Journal of Translational Medicine* 13, no. 33 (2015): 1–4.

38. S. H. Gonzalez, "The Cowpox Controversy: Memory and the Politics of Public Health in Cuba," *Bulletin of the History of Medicine* 92, no. 1 (2018): 110–40.

39. Jouve Martin, *Black Doctors*, 60–94.

40. Cueto, *Medicine and Public Health*, 48.

41. Cueto, 48.

42. Warren, *Colonial Peru*, 104.

CHAPTER II

1. Ivan Jaksic, *Andrés Bello: Scholarship and Nation-Building in Nineteenth-Century Latin America* (Cambridge: Cambridge University Press, 2001), 11–13.

2. For a good analysis of the early life of Bello, see Jaksic, *Andrés Bello*.

3. *British and Foreign Medico-chirurgical Review*, vol. 45, 315.

4. A. von Humboldt, *Political Essay on the Kingdom of New Spain*, vol. 1, A Critical Edition (Chicago: University of Chicago Press, 2019).

5. *British and Foreign Medico-chirurgical Review*, vol. 45, 319.

6. *British and Foreign Medico-chirurgical Review*, vol. 45, 319.

7. Moore, *History and Practice of Vaccination*, 287.

8. Frederick Ober, *Popular History of Mexico* (Boston: Estes and Lauriat, 1894), 404 and 408.

9. Alamán in volume 1 of his work mentions Balmis in a brief sentence, surrounded by a paragraph-long description of Iturrigaray's efforts. See Lucas Alamán, *Historia de Mexico, Vol. I* (Mexico City: Victoriano Agueros, 1883), 137–38.

10. Warren, *Colonial Peru*, 106.

11. Quoted in Warren, 106.

12. Alessandro Malaspina, *The Malaspina Expedition Journal* (London: Hakluyt Society, 2004), 178.

13. Marcos Cueto, "History of Public Health in Latin America," *Oxford Research Encyclopedia of Global Public Health* (New York: Oxford University Press, 2019).

14. Frederick Ober, *Young Folk's History of Mexico* (Boston: D. Lothrop, 1883), 298.

15. Riccardo Liberatore, "The Balmis Expedition," *East* 57 (December 28, 2014).

16. Elena de Lorenzo Alvarez, "Notas sobre la renovacion de la poesia propuesta por los ilustrados" in *Homenaje a José María Martínez Cachero*, vol. 3, ed. José María Martínez Cachero (Oviedo: Universidad de Oviedo, 2000), 70.

17. Ober, *History of Mexico*, 410.

18. "Mexican President Asks Spain to Apologize for Actions During Conquest," *Reuters*, March 25, 2019.

19. *British and Foreign Medico-chirurgical Review*, vol. 44, 328.

20. William White, *The Story of a Great Delusion in a Series of Matter-of-Fact Chapters* (London: Allen, 1885), 403.

21. Lord Byron, *Don Juan*, canto 1, sts. 129 and 130.

22. S. F. Cook, "Francisco Xavier Balmis and the Introduction of Vaccination to Latin America, Part 1," *Bulletin of the History of Medicine* 11, no. 5 (May 1942): 543–60 and "Francisco Xavier Balmis and the Introduction of Vaccination to Latin America, Part 2," *Bulletin of the History of Medicine* 12, no. 1 (June 1942): 70–101.

23. Quoted in de Yraola, *Expedición de la vacuna*, 90.

CONCLUSION

1. Data as per the CDC, "Estimated Flu-Related Illnesses, Medical Visits, Hospitalizations, and Deaths in the United States—2017–2018 Flu Season," https://www.cdc.gov/flu/about/burden/2017-2018.htm and "All Injuries," https://www.cdc.gov/nchs/fastats/injury.htm. Gun deaths exclude suicides.

2. John W. Dietrich, "The Politics of PEPFAR: The President's Emergency Plan for AIDS Relief," *Ethics and International Affairs* 21, no. 3 (Fall 2007): 277–92.

3. John S. Santelli, "Abstinence Promotion Under PEPFAR: The Shifting Focus of HIV Prevention for Youth," *Global Public Health* 8, no. 1 (2013): 1–12.

4. Kate Winksall, Laura K. Beres, Elizabeth Hill, Benjamin Chigozie Mbakwem, and Oby Obyerodhyambo, "Making Sense of Abstinence: Social Representations in Young Africans' HIV-Related Narratives from Six Countries," *Culture, Health and Sexuality* 13, no. 8 (September 2011): 945–59.

5. Edward C. Green, "Uganda's HIV Prevention Success: The Role of Sexual Behavior Change and the National Response," *AIDS Behavior* 10, no. 4 (July 2006): 335–46.

Index

Aguilar, Rafael Maria, 148, 149, 151, 152

Alfonso X of Castile, 49, 50, 193

Alfonso XI of Castile, 9, 50

Amar, Antonio Jose, 132

Antonine Plague, 8, 25

Argentina, 33, 41, 78, 118, 138, 140

Aztec, 18, 29, 34, 36, 59, 151

bartonellosis, 29, 33

begonia, 75

Bello, Andres, 95, 181

Black Legend, 4, 28, 187-188, 190, 197

Black Plague, 9-10, 13

Bogota, 90, 95, 118, 129, 131, 133, 134, 138, 165, 179,

Bourbon Reforms, 40, 55-56, 73-74, 186, 195

Brazil, 36, 37, 48, 174, 176

Canary Islands, 59, 92, 110-112, 115, 124, 169, 183

Caracas, 76, 90, 116, 118, 130, 155, 162, 165, 179

Caribbean, 35-41, 63-64, 73, 89, 95, 111, 113, 128-129, 165, 185

Cartagena, 38, 93-95, 98, 118, 128-131, 133, 179

Catholic Church, 2, 46, 48-50, 88, 91, 98, 99, 105, 126, 132, 133, 150, 179, 188, 193, 196,

Charles II, 24, 55, 91,

Charles III, 3, 56, 58, 61, 64-65, 67, 72, 82, 96, 148, 153, 177, 188, 195

Charles IV, 5, 58, 82, 91-93, 95-96, 100, 105, 109, 114, 117, 127, 132, 140, 148, 156-158, 176-177, 181, 183-186, 188, 191, 196

Charles V, 14

Chile, 32-33, 36, 61, 67, 88, 134, 136, 139-143, 166-167

China, 25, 40, 62, 67, 143-146, 152-153, 156, 174, 198

Columbus, Christopher, 13, 28, 35, 143, 194

Comuneros Uprising, 40

Cordoba, 11-12, 53, 184, 193

Cortes, Hernan, 29-32, 34, 36, 48, 131

Crespo, Angel, 104, 147, 149, 156

Cuba, 38, 39, 59, 64, 118-119, 128, 163-165, 178

Cuzco, 139-140

Cyprian Plague, 8

de Aviles, Gabriel, 136

de Castro, Ramon, 113

de Galvez, Bernardo, 82

de Mayorga, Martin, 80, 82

de Muro, Salvador de Jose, 119, 163

de Ochoa, Ramon, 104-105

diphtheria, 18, 54

dysentery, 23, 31, 60, 133

Enlightenment, 2-5, 43-57

Esparragosa, Narcisco, 94, 121

Ferdinand I of Aragon, 11

Ferdinand II of Aragon, 19
Ferdinand III of Aragon, 55
Ferdinand VI, 56, 92
Ferdinand VI, 157
Flores, Jose, 86-88, 94, 96-101, 104, 112,
    121, 125, 162, 186
Folch, Jose Solis, 89
Francisco Hernandez Expedition, 30,
    58

Grajales, Julian, 104-105, 128, 139-141, 167
Guatemala, 64, 80, 86-87, 94, 96-97,
    120-121, 155

Habsburgs, 14, 19-24, 55, 78, 91, 166, 193
Havana, 39, 56, 74, 94, 119-122, 155, 163-
    164
Hospital of Amor de Dios, 74, 82,
Huey Cocoliztli, 29-30, 60

Inca, 28, 32-33, 137, 139
Isabella I of Castile, 19-21
Isabella II, 176
Iturrigaray, Jose de, 94, 122-125, 147,
    157-158, 178

Jenner, Edward, 68-77
Jesty, Benjamin, 69-70
Jews in Spain, 10, 13, 44-45
Joanna the Mad, 21-22
Justinianic Plague, 8
Lima, 61, 95, 134, 136-141, 186
Lisbon Plague of 1432, 11
Lopez-Pavon Expedition, 61-62

Macau, 152-154
Malaspina Expedition, 65-66, 82, 148,
    186

Manila, 120, 145-150, 153, 168, 183
Martin of Aragon, 11
Matlazanhuatl Epidemic, 39, 79
Mendinueta, Pedro, 78, 90-91, 132
Mexico, 30, 32, 36, 39, 41, 48, 57, 60,
    63-64, 74-76, 79-88, 94, 116, 120-128,
    134, 145, 147, 158-162, 178, 183-184
Mompox, 130-131
Morel, Esteban, 41, 80-81, 99
Mutis Expedition, 62-63, 90-91, 133

New Granada, 40, 62, 74, 76, 89-91,
    95-96, 117-118, 129-132, 135-140, 165,
    177, 179, 181, 182, 195
Nueva Planta Decrees, 55

O'Gorman, Miguel, 41, 136
O'Sullivan, Daniel, 75-76
Oller, Francisco, 113-117, 162, 177, 185

Parker, Janet, 1
Pedro IV of Castile, 10
Peru, 61, 67, 83, 88, 90, 97, 118, 134,
    136-140, 165, 167, 177-178, 185, 195
Peter IV of Aragon, 10
Philip II, 14-15, 22, 59-60, 73, 92
Philip III, 23,
Philip IV, 23
Philip V, 55-56, 92,
Philippines, 65-66, 111-112, 125, 143-154,
    159, 167-168, 183-184, 198
Pizarro, Francisco, 33
Porcell, Juan Tomas, 54
Puerto Rico, 36, 112-113, 116-119, 121, 125,
    155, 162-164, 167, 180, 185

Real Protomedicato, 73
Reconquista, 8, 11, 26, 53, 73, 194

Renaissance, 11, 52, 59, 99, 193

Salamanca, School of, 54, 57
Salvany, Jose, 104-105, 115-118, 128-141, 159, 165, 177-179, 186, 197-198
Sesse Expedition, 63-64, 82
Smallpox Epidemic of 1779, 41, 79, 81, 85-86
Smallpox Epidemic of 1802, 93-96, 113
Spanish Armada, 14-16, 38
syphilis, 13-14, 26, 52, 75, 82, 176, 194

Talamanca, Miguel, 76, 82-84
typhus, 12, 14, 16-17, 26, 29, 32, 38, 82-83, 85, 194

variolation, 40-42, 48, 57, 70-71, 80-84, 86-88, 90, 97, 99-100, 113, 122, 150, 153, 160, 170, 172, 174, 196
Varna, Nicolas, 75
Venezuela, 31, 95, 128, 131, 179
Virgin of Guadalupe, 40
von Humboldt, Alexander, 76, 183

War of Jenkins' Ear, 37-39

yellow fever, 34, 38-39, 64, 74, 76, 86-87, 120, 123, 133, 163-165, 179, 195

Zendal, Isabel, 106-107, 110, 145, 159, 190
Zulaibar, Juan Antonio, 149-150

About the Author

DAVID PETRIELLO received his doctorate from St. John's University. He has authored a dozen books and articles on subjects ranging from disease and civilization to American conservative politics to military history. His most notable works are *Bacteria and Bayonets*, *A Pestilence on Pennsylvania Avenue*, and *The Republican Party and the Growth of China*. He teaches at Caldwell University in New Jersey.

Printed in the USA
CPSIA information can be obtained
at www.ICGtesting.com
CBHW030751061224
18505CB00008B/551

9 780875 658575